Modern
Dental
Assisting

WORKBOOK

Hazel O. Torres, CDA, RDA, RDAEF, MA
Ann Ehrlich, CDA, MA
Doni Bird, CDA, RDH, MA
Ellen Dietz, CDA, AAS, BS

Modern Dental Assisting
WORKBOOK

fifth edition

W.B. SAUNDERS COMPANY
A Division of Harcourt Brace & Company
Philadelphia London Toronto Montreal Sydney Tokyo

W.B. Saunders Company
A Division of
Harcourt Brace & Company
The Curtis Center
Independence Square West
Philadelphia, Pa 19106

Workbook to accompany Modern Dental Assisting, 5/e   ISBN 0-7216-5056-2

Printed in the United States of America.

Last digit is the print number: 9   8   7   6   5   4   3   2

Workbook to Accompany

Modern Dental Assisting, 5th ed

Table of Contents

Introduction to the Workbook to Accompany Modern Dental Assisting, 5th edition

To the Student:

This workbook is designed to help you master the information and skills presented in the textbook. To help you understand and apply the content of the chapter, the workbook includes learning objectives, exercises, and competency sheets for each chapter.

Because this text is used throughout the United States, and in many other countries, the authors have included extended function procedures that are legally assigned to dental assistants in many states. If any of these procedures are **not legal** in your state, you should not perform them. Contact your State Board of Dentistry for details as to what is, and is not, legal in your state.

There are regional and personal preferences in performing many procedures. Those presented here represent one commonly accepted technique; however your instructor or employer may prefer that a different, and equally acceptable, technique be used.

The discussion of OSHA regulations and CDC guidelines, which were current when this book was published, apply across the United States. However, these too are subject to change. In your studies, you must learn and follow the most recent regulations and guidelines that are applicable in the state where you are employed.

Learning Objectives

A learning objective is a statement of what the student should be able to do upon successful completion of that chapter. In the limited space available it would be impossible to include all of the objectives for all the chapters, and your instructor may add more objectives for each chapter.

Exercises

The exercise portion of each chapter includes 25 questions. These are intended to help you study, interact with, and better understand the information presented in the corresponding chapter of the textbook. Please take time to work through them carefully. The correct answer to each question can be found in the textbook.

Competency Sheets

A competency is the skill expected of an entry level dental assistant. Competency sheets, which are included with chapters when applicable, give you opportunities to practice until you have mastered that skill. A space on the form allows for at least three different evaluations. The first time you may wish to evaluate your performance. The second time you might ask a class-mate to give you feedback. When you feel comfortable with that skill, the evaluator should be your instructor or clinic supervisor.

The ability to objectively evaluate your performance is an important skill to develop. Once you are working in a dental practice many of the important tasks assigned to you are performed without direct supervision. In this situation *you* are responsible for maintaining your skills and for the quality of your work.

For those competencies that require instruments and materials, the second page has space to list the required items. Developing this list provides valuable experience in planning the supplies that must be gathered or prepared before performing that procedure. The icons used on the instrumentation list are the same as those used throughout the textbook.

These are from left to right: *examination gloves, protective mask* and *protective eyewear, basic setup, local anesthetic,* and *dental dam.*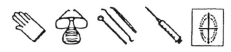

Conclusion

It is the hope of the authors that this workbook will be a meaningful aid as you prepare to enter the profession of dental assisting. Best wishes from:

Hazel O. Torres

Ann Ehrlich

Doni Bird

Ellen Dietz

Competency 3 - 1 *Identifying Anatomic Landmarks of the Face (1)*

Performance Objective: When working with another student, or through the use of a mannikin, or photograph, the student will identify the landmarks of the face as listed below.

Note: If working with a person, the student will point but not touch the face.

Evaluator #1 (Name/date) _____

Evaluator #2 (Name/date) _____

Evaluator #3 (Name/date) _____

Check box if step was performed correctly.	1st	2nd	3rd
1. Identified the ala of the nose.	☐	☐	☐
2. Identified the inner canthus of the eye.	☐	☐	☐
3. Identified the outer canthus of the eye.	☐	☐	☐
4. Identified the commissures of the lips.	☐	☐	☐
5. Identified the midline (midsagittal plane).	☐	☐	☐

Notes:

Competency 3 - 2 *Identifying Anatomic Landmarks of the Face (2)*

Performance Objective: When working with another student, or through the use of a mannikin or photograph, the student will identify the landmarks of the face as listed below.

Note: If working with a person, the student will point but not touch the face.

Evaluator #1 (Name/date) _____

Evaluator #2 (Name/date) _____

Evaluator #3 (Name/date) _____

Check box if step was performed correctly.	1st	2nd	3rd
1. Identified the nasion.	☐	☐	☐
2. Identified the philtrum.	☐	☐	☐
3. Identified the tragus of the ear.	☐	☐	☐
4. Identified the vermilion border.	☐	☐	☐
5. Identified the zygomatic arch	☐	☐	☐

Notes:

14

Competency 5 - 1 *Identifying Types of Teeth*

Performance Objective: Given five teeth, the student will identify each tooth as to the type, and classify each as to whether it is an anterior or a posterior tooth.

Note: This is an entry level skill. Students are expected to continue to improve their skills until they can identify any tooth in the permanent or primary dentition and state whether it comes from the maxillary or mandibular arch.

Important: *The instructor will supply the teeth to be identified. These will be from a typodont or sterilized extracted teeth and will be lettered A, B, C, D, and E. No additional instrumentation is required for this procedure.*

Evaluator #1 (Name/date) _____

Evaluator #2 (Name/date) _____

Evaluator #3 (Name/date) _____

Check box if step was performed correctly.	1st	2nd	3rd
1. **Tooth A:** Identified type of tooth.	☐	☐	☐
2. **Tooth A:** Identified it correctly as an anterior or a posterior tooth.	☐	☐	☐
3. **Tooth B:** Identified type of tooth.	☐	☐	☐
4. **Tooth B:** Identified it correctly as an anterior or a posterior tooth.	☐	☐	☐
5. **Tooth C:** Identified type of tooth.	☐	☐	☐
6. **Tooth C:** Identified it correctly as an anterior or a posterior tooth.	☐	☐	☐
7. **Tooth D:** Identified type of tooth.	☐	☐	☐
8. **Tooth D:** Identified it correctly as an anterior or a posterior tooth.	☐	☐	☐
9. **Tooth E:** Identified type of tooth.	☐	☐	☐
10. **Tooth E:** Identified it correctly as an anterior or a posterior tooth.	☐	☐	☐

Notes:

Competency 5 - 2 *Identifying Permanent Teeth*

Performance Objective: The student will identify each tooth as to the type of tooth it is, and state whether it is a maxillary or mandibular tooth.

Important: *The instructor will supply five sterilized extracted teeth, or typodont teeth with roots. These will be labeled A, B, C, D, E. No additional instrumentation is required for this procedure.*

Evaluator #1 (Name/date) _____

Evaluator #2 (Name/date) _____

Evaluator #3 (Name/date) _____

Check box if step was performed correctly.	1st	2nd	3rd
1. **Tooth A:** Stated the type of tooth.	☐	☐	☐
2. **Tooth A:** Identified it as a maxillary or mandibular tooth.	☐	☐	☐
3. **Tooth B:** Stated the type of tooth.	☐	☐	☐
4. **Tooth B:** Identified it as a maxillary or mandibular tooth.	☐	☐	☐
5. **Tooth C:** Stated the type of tooth.	☐	☐	☐
6. **Tooth C:** Identified it as a maxillary or mandibular tooth.	☐	☐	☐
7. **Tooth D:** Stated the type of tooth.	☐	☐	☐
8. **Tooth D:** Identified it as a maxillary or mandibular tooth.	☐	☐	☐
9. **Tooth E:** Stated the type of tooth.	☐	☐	☐
10. **Tooth E:** Identified it as a maxillary or mandibular tooth.	☐	☐	☐

Notes:

Chapter 6:
Preventive Dentistry and Nutrition

Student's Name _____

Learning Objectives

Upon completion of this chapter, the student should be able to:

☐   Describe how dental decay occurs and discuss the role of cariogenic foods in dental caries.

☐   Identify the key nutrients, describe their primary functions, define empty calories, and discuss the use of the Food Pyramid as a means of evaluating dietary intake.

☐   List the four key components in preventive dentistry and discuss the roles of systemic and topical fluorides in preventive dentistry.

☐   Describe cheilitis, demineralization, glossitis, remineralization, and scurvy.

☐   Describe the components of plaque, its formation, and patterns of accumulation on the teeth.

☐   Demonstrate personal oral hygiene, including use of a disclosing agent, brushing, flossing, and repeated disclosing.

☐   Demonstrate providing personal oral hygiene instruction to a patient.

Exercises

Circle the letter next to the correct answer.

1. The occlusal surfaces of the teeth are brushed with a small _____ motion.
   a. back and forth
   b. circular
   c. scrubbing
   d. A and B

2. When using a disclosing agent at home, the patient should be instructed to _____ .
   a. rub the excess on his lips to disclose any lesions
   b. spit the excess into a sink with running water
   c. swallow the excess

3. _____ vitamins are easily destroyed during food preparation.
   a. Fat-soluble
   b. Water soluble

4. The most effective way to remove plaque from proximal tooth surfaces is by _____ .
   a. flossing
   b. oral irrigation
   c. rinsing vigorously
   d. toothbrushing

5. Each gram of fat contains _____ calories.
   a. 4
   b. 7
   c. 9
   d. 15

6. _____ plaque develops on tooth surfaces, restorations, appliances, and dentures.
   a. Epithelium-associated
   b. Subgingival
   c. Supragingival
   d. Tooth-associated

7. When brushing the lingual surfaces of the anterior teeth, the head of the toothbrush is placed in a _____ position.
   a. horizontal
   b. vertical

8. The only nutrients that can make new cells and rebuild body tissues are _____.
   a. carbohydrates
   b. fats
   c. minerals
   d. proteins

9. Once plaque has been thoroughly removed, it takes about _____ hours for it to form again.
   a. 6
   b. 12
   c. 24
   d. 36

10. Fluoridated toothpaste is a source of _____ fluoride.
    a. systemic
    b. topical

11. In water fluoridation, the ratio of fluoride to water is _____ .
   a. 3 drops per gallon
   b. 1 part per consumer
   c. 1 part per thousand
   d. 1 part per million

12. Only energy, and no other nutrients, is provided by _____ .
   a. carbohydrates
   b. empty calories
   c. fats

13. _____ plaque contains predominately, but not exclusively, motile gram-negative organisms.
   a. Attached subgingival
   b. Epithelium-associated subgingival
   c. Supragingival

14. Sticky sugary refined products are _____ cariogenic than complex carbohydrates.
   a. less
   b. more

15. The infant fed only breast milk usually receives _____ quantities of fluoride.
   a. excessive
   b. optimal
   c. insufficient

16. During remineralization, _____ found in saliva work together to replace some of the minerals that have been lost.
   a. calcium and fluoride
   b. calcium, fluoride, and phosphate
   c. iron, fluoride, and phosphate
   d. None of the above, fluorides work alone

17. Excess systemic fluoride intake is _____ .
   a. excreted by the kidneys
   b. stored in the bones
   c. stored in the teeth
   d. B and C

18. _____ is a condition that affects the gingiva and is the result of a severe vitamin C deficiency.
   a. Angular cheilitis
   b. Glossitis
   c. Scurvy

19. A young child should be instructed to _____ a fluoride containing toothpaste.
    a. avoid swallowing
    b. swallow only small quantities of
    c. swish and swallow with

20. If a patient has badly decayed teeth, it _____ possible for re-mineralization to reverse the decay process.
    a. is
    b. is not

21. The patient learns most effectively when he _____ .
    a. feels safe and accepted
    b. is actively involved
    c. recognizes that he has a problem to be solved
    d. A, B, and C

21. Topical fluoride rinses are recommended for high-risk patients. These include _____ .
    a. nursing mothers
    b. patients with a high caries rate
    c. patients with a reduced flow of saliva
    d. B and C

22. As a precautionary measure, it is recommended that no more than _____ mg. of sodium fluoride supplements be dispensed at one time.
    a. 100
    b. 223
    c. 264
    d. 296

23. Prolonged exposure to excessive fluoride may cause _____ .
    a. dental decay
    b. dental fluorosis
    c. periodontal disease
    d. A, B, and C

24. _____ is a colorless, translucent film composed of complex sugar-protein molecules that are a product of the saliva.
    a. Acquired pellicle
    c. Subgingival plaque
    d. Supragingival plaque

25. Prescription fluoride rinses are designed to be used _____ .
    a. daily
    b. once a week

28

Competency 6 - 1 Demonstrating Personal Oral Hygiene

Performance Objective: The student will demonstrate his or her personal oral hygiene skills by using disclosing solution, then flossing and brushing. Upon completion, disclosing solution is applied again to demonstrate that all plaque has been removed.

Important: *The student will need disclosing solution (or tablets), a toothbrush, toothpaste (optional), dental floss, and other aids as indicated by the instructor.*

Evaluator #1 (Name/date) _____

Evaluator #2 (Name/date) _____

Evaluator #3 (Name/date) _____

Check box if step was performed correctly.	1st	2nd	3rd
1. Used disclosing agent to disclose plaque.	☐	☐	☐
2. Brushed teeth without trauma to the gingiva.	☐	☐	☐
3. Used floss removing remaining plaque without trauma to the gingiva.	☐	☐	☐
4. Used other aids as indicated by the instructor.	☐	☐	☐
5. Repeated use of disclosing agent indicated that all plaque has been removed.	☐	☐	☐

Notes:

Competency 6 - 2 *Teaching Personal Oral Hygiene Skills*

Performance Objective: The student will demonstrate the use of disclosing solution (or tablets), toothbrushing, and dental floss to remove plaque without injury to the gingiva.

Note: Gloves are not worn during this procedure because the assistant does not place his or her hands in the patient's mouth.

Important: *The student may use a large model and toothbrush for the demonstration. The "patient" should be supplied with disclosing solution or tablets, a new toothbrush and dental floss.*

Evaluator #1 (Name/date) _____

Evaluator #2 (Name/date) _____

Evaluator #3 (Name/date) _____

Check box if step was performed correctly.	1st	2nd	3rd
1. Gathered appropriate supplies.	☐	☐	☐
2. Explained the procedure to the patient.	☐	☐	☐
3. Explained the use of the disclosing agent and instructed the patient how to use it.	☐	☐	☐
4. Observed patient during use of the disclosing agent and made constructive suggestions as necessary.	☐	☐	☐
5. Instructed patient in toothbrushing..	☐	☐	☐
6. Observed patient during toothbrushing and made constructive suggestions as necessary.	☐	☐	☐
7. Instructed patient in the use of dental floss.	☐	☐	☐
8. Observed patient during flossing and made constructive suggestions as necessary.	☐	☐	☐
9. Had patient reapply disclosing agent.	☐	☐	☐
10. Congratulated and encouraged the patient when efforts were successful.	☐	☐	☐

Notes:

30

Chapter 7:
Psychology and Communication

Student's Name _____

Learning Objectives

Upon completion of this chapter, the student should be able to:

❐   Differentiate between psychotic, neurotic, and normal behavior.

❐   Discuss understanding patient behavior in terms of: factors affecting behavior, fear, emotional elements, phobias, and patient responses.

❐   Identify the following coping mechanisms: affiliation, control of the situation, deployment, procrastination, rationalization, rehearsal, and repression.

❐   Differentiate between verbal and nonverbal communication and describe how we communicate nonverbally.

❐   Describe the difference between closed-ended and open-ended questions.

❐   List at least four causes of stress that may occur in the dental office and describe at least four recommended forms of stress reduction.

Exercises

Circle the letter next to the correct answer.

1. The causes of stress in the dental office may include _____ .
    a.   appointment overbooking
    b.   lack of good communication
    c.   multiple tasks required simultaneously
    d.   A, B, and C

2. _____ is an example of a psychosis characterized by delusions of persecution.
    a.   Anxiety
    b.   A dental phobia
    c.   Paranoia
    d.   Schizophrenia

3. Rationalization _____ the process of making plausible excuses or reasons for implausible behavior.
    a.   is
    b.   is not

4. A phobia _____ .
   a. is a multiple personality disorder
   b. is a neurotic state
   c. prevents otherwise normal patients from seeking treatment
   d. B and C

5. Important factors that may influence a patient's reactions to dental treatment include _____ .
   a. attitudes
   b. current life situation
   c. previous dental experience
   d. A, B, and C

6. For many patients, _____ pain is the greatest cause for distress.
   a. actual
   b. the expectation of

7. Subjective fears are based on _____ .
   a. attitudes and concerns
   b. feelings that have developed through the suggestions of others
   c. the patient's personal experience
   d. A and B

8. Stress associated with employment may be reduced by _____ .
   a. engaging in regular exercise
   b. living a balanced life
   c. setting realistic expectations
   d. A, B, and C

9. Patients for whom the mere suggestion of a routine dental visit brings overwhelming sensations of panic and terror are termed _____ .
   a. dental phobics
   b. dental schizophrenics
   c. passive aggressive
   d. psychotic

10. Reasons for distributing a practice newsletter to patients include _____ .
    a. advertising seasonal special rates
    b. informing patients about technological and treatment advances
    c. keeping patients in touch with the doctor and staff
    d. B and C

11. Repression _____ the temporary unconscious forgetting of things that produce tension and/or pain.
    a. is
    b. is not

12. A compulsive personality disorder is characterized by _____ .
    a. personal insecurity
    b. doubt
    c. excessive conscientiousness
    d. all of the above

13. Deployment is _____ .
    a. an effective coping mechanism in the dental setting
    b. avoiding an upsetting situation by postponing facing it
    c. the turning of attention away from an unpleasant stimulus
    d. A and C

14. _____ is the act of mentally going through a situation before it actually occurs.
    a. Affiliation
    b. Deployment
    c. Procrastination
    d. Rehearsal

15. Communication is _____ .
    a. an important part of the assistant's job
    b. both verbal and nonverbal
    c. consists of sending and receiving the same message
    d. A, B, and C

16. Nonverbal communication may include _____ .
    a. actions
    b. attitudes
    c. body language
    d. A, B, and C

17. When speaking to the patient, the dental assistant _____ use technical dental language and jargon.
    a. should
    b. should not

18. *"Mr. Harris, is next Monday at 9 A.M. convenient for you?"* is an example of a/an _____ question.
    a. closed-ended
    b. open-ended

19. It has been estimated that _____ percent of all spoken words are never heard.
    a. 20
    b. 50
    c. 75
    d. 90

20. A good listener _____ .
    a. concentrates on what the person is actually saying
    b. does not let his/her mind wander
    c. prepares his or her answer
    d. A and B

21. Coping mechanisms are a/an _____ .
    a. indication of a neurotic phobia
    b. symptom of psychotic behavior
    c. useful way of handling an uncomfortable situation

22. When addressing an adult patient for the first time, it is appropriate to _____ .
    a. address the patient as "Mr.," "Mrs.," Miss" or "Ms."
    b. ask the patient how he or she prefers to be addressed
    c. make up a nickname for the patient and enter it on the chart
    d. A and B

23. When a patient appears to be angry or upset, the assistant should _____ .
    a. argue with the patient
    b. calm the patient down by listening and remaining approachable
    c. tell the patient the doctor is too busy to talk to him or her
    d. B and C

24. Professional communications sent out of the office should _____ .
    a. be carefully and neatly typed
    b. be free of typographical and spelling errors
    c. reflect a positive image of the practice
    d. A, B, and C

25. Techniques used successfully to treat dental phobics include _____ .
    a. guided imagery
    b. progressive muscle relaxation
    c. systematic desensitization
    d. A, B, and C

Chapter 8:
The Special Patient

Student's Name _____

Learning Objectives

Upon completion of this chapter, the student should be able to:

☐ Describe the child's development through infancy, early childhood, preschool age and grade school age, as well as differentiate between chronological, mental, and emotional age.

☐ Describe management techniques and precautions when treating the pregnant patient.

☐ Identify at least three special dental problems faced by the older patient.

☐ Describe the role of the dental team in detecting and reporting suspected cases of child, spouse, or geriatric abuse.

☐ Discuss the three major areas in which the assistant aids in providing dental care for a handicapped patient.

☐ Explain the four degrees of intellectual impairment associated with mental retardation.

☐ List at least three problems afflicting infants born with a cleft palate.

☐ Describe the special needs of dental patients with Alzheimer's disease, arthritis, asthma, cardiovascular disorders, diabetes, Down syndrome, epilepsy, muscular dystrophy, and severe kidney disease.

Exercises

Circle the letter next to the correct answer.

1. A child's _____ age refers to his level of intellectual capacity and development.
   a. chronological
   b. emotional
   c. mental
   d. physical

2. In most cases, _____ diabetes can be controlled through diet and oral medication(s).
   a. Type I
   b. Type II

3. The patient with _____ may have dental abnormalities such as small peg-shaped teeth, forward position of the mandible, and a large, fissured tongue.
   a. cerebral palsy
   b. cleft palate
   c. Down syndrome
   d. epilepsy

4. When speaking to a patient who is hearing impaired, the dental assistant should _____ .
   a. shout
   b. speak slowly
   c. stand where he can see your lip movements
   d. B and C

5. The childhood stage from ages _____ years has been described as the "out-of-bounds" age.
   a. birth to 2
   b. 2 to 4
   c. 4 to 6
   d. 6 to 12

6. The Americans with Disabilities Act provides disabled people with access to equal goods and services.
   a. true
   b. false

7. Oral manifestations of _____ include acetone breath, dehydration of oral soft tissues, and delayed healing.
   a. asthma
   b. diabetes
   c. epilepsy
   d. muscular dystrophy

8. Spasticity and athetosis are common types of _____ .
   a. arteriosclerosis
   b. cerebral palsy
   c. Down syndrome
   d. muscular dystrophy

9. _____, which is used to control epileptic seizures, causes hyperplasia of the gingival tissues.
   a. Dilantin
   b. Dyslexia
   c. Insulin
   d. Vitamin C

10. Symptoms of possible child abuse include _____ .
    a. broken teeth
    b. facial bruises
    c. swelling of the facial structures
    d. A, B, and C

11. _____ is a chronic systemic disease affecting the connective tissues and joints in which the joints are swollen, deformed, and painful.
    a. Osteoarthritis
    b. Rheumatoid arthritis

12. When abuse is suspected in a child patient, the assistant should report this to the _____ .
    a. dentist
    b. office manager
    c. nearest Social Services agency

13. A/An _____ year-old child has all of his primary teeth and is usually ready for his or her first dental visit.
    a. one-
    b. two-
    c. three-
    d. four-

14. During an asthmatic attack, the patient will _____ .
    a. complain of chest pain
    b. faint
    c. make a wheezing sound as he breathes
    d. sweat profusely

15. A pregnant patient _____ .
    a. can usually safely undergo routine dental care
    b. can safely receive treatment only during the first trimester
    c. should receive emergency treatment only until after delivery

16. A cleft palate patient may wear an appliance known as a/an _____, which blocks the opening in the palate.
    a. obturator
    b. oral brace
    c. palatoscope
    d. shunt

17. Patients with known cardiovascular disorders should be treated with local anesthesia _____ epinephrine.
    a. with
    b. without

18. A mildly retarded patient _____ .
    a. can usually cooperate during treatment
    b. must receive treatment under general anesthesia

19. An older patient may suffer from _____ , which is a dry mouth.
    a. angina
    b. hyperplasia
    c. xerostomia

20. While a patient with a pacemaker is in the office, avoid use of the _____ .
    a. computer
    b. high-speed handpiece
    c. ultrasonic scaler
    d. B and C

21. A _____ seizure lasts no longer than 30 seconds.
    a. grand mal
    b. petit mal

22. _____ is a chronic lung disorder in which the patient has ongoing and increasing difficulty in breathing.
    a. Asthma
    b. Emphysema
    c. Multiple sclerosis
    d. Muscular dystrophy

23. A diabetic patient should be treated with _____ prior to dental appointments
    a. antibiotics
    b. anticoagulants
    c. antihistamines
    d. None of the above

24. _____ is a progressive chronic degenerative disease of cognitive function.
    a. Alzheimer's disease
    b. Cerebral palsy
    c. Mental retardation
    d. Muscular dystrophy

25. The kidney disease patient may have a tendency to hemorrhage because he is usually given _____ both during and after dialysis.
    a. antibiotics
    b. anticoagulants
    c. coagulants

38

Chapter 9:
Medical Emergencies

Student's Name _____

Learning Objectives

Upon completion of this chapter, the student should be able to:

☐   Describe the types of medical emergencies that may be encountered in a dental office and discuss the role of staff members in managing these emergencies.

☐   Identify the supplies found in a dental office emergency kit and state the purpose of each item.

☐   Describe the basic emergency management of anaphylactic reactions, cardiac distress, choking, diabetic emergencies, hemorrhage, seizures, shock, and stroke.

☐   Demonstrate taking and recording vital signs.

☐   Demonstrate treatment for syncope and postural hypotension.

Exercises

Circle the letter next to the correct answer.

1. Episodes of spasmodic suffocating chest pain that are relieved by the administration of nitroglycerin are characteristic of _____ .
   a. angina pectoris
   b. diabetic acidosis
   c. hypoglycemia
   d. myocardial infarction

2. During an epileptic seizure, the patient should be _____ .
   a. placed in a prone position
   b. positioned with the feet elevated

3. Tannic acid, which is found in tea, aids in _____ .
   a. clot formation
   b. relieving pain
   c. stopping hemorrhaging
   d. A and C

4. When performing abdominal thrusts, the hands are positioned firmly _____ the xiphoid of the sternum.
    a. above
    b. below
    c. on

5. A patient experiencing _____ will breathe in short, gasping inspirations with long, wheezing expirations.
    a. a bronchospasm
    b. an epileptic seizure
    c. hyperventilation
    d. syncope

6. The purpose of an ammonia inhalant is to _____ .
    a. cause the patient to inhale quickly
    b. dilate the bronchioles
    c. relieve spasms of the pharynx
    d. none of the above

7. The fingers are placed along the side of the patient's neck to check the _____ pulse.
    a. carotid
    b. radial

8. In a severe allergic reaction _____ .
    a. an antihistamine may be administered
    b. epinephrine may be administered
    c. the patient is placed in a supine position with the feet elevated
    d. A, B, and C

9. When taking and recording blood pressure, the lowest pressure is the _____ pressure and this number is recorded _____ .
    a. diastolic   first
    b. diastolic   last
    c. systolic   first
    d. systolic   last

10. The unconscious hypoglycemia patient is treated by _____ .
    a. forcing orange juice into his mouth
    b. performing abdominal thrusts
    c. smearing liquid sugar on the oral mucosa
    d. A and B

40

11. When the diabetic's breath smells like fruit, he is probably suffering from
    _____ and requires immediate medical attention.
    a. diabetic acidosis
    b. hypoglycemia
    c. insulin shock
    d. B or C

12. When establishing an airway, a finger sweep is performed only on a/an
    _____ patient.
    a. conscious
    b. unconscious

13. The pulse is counted for _____ seconds and then multiplied by two.
    a. 15
    b. 30
    c. 60

14. If the patient is in respiratory failure _____ .
    a. breathing will be labored
    b. CPR should be started immediately
    c. there will be little or no movement of the chest
    d. B and C

15. If a patient indicates that he is choking, _____ should be started
    immediately.
    a. abdominal thrusts (Heimlich maneuver)
    b. administering oxygen
    c. CPR
    d. rescue breathing

16. During rescue breathing for a child, the inflation rate should be
    _____ times per minute.
    a. 10
    b. 15
    c. 20
    d. 30

17. If the patient becomes pale, perspires, and feels dizzy, he is probably suffering
    from _____ .
    a. anaphylaxis
    b. hyperventilation
    c. syncope
    d. B or C

18. No heart beat or pulse is a diagnostic sign of _____ .
    a. cardiac arrest
    b. respiratory failure

19. The heart attack patient may complain of pain in the _____ .
    a. left arm
    b. mandible
    c. sternum
    d. A, B and C

20. The resuscitation mask placed on the oxygen source _____ the same as the mask used to administer nitrous oxide-oxygen sedation.
    a. is
    b. is not

21. A local anesthetic overdose is treated first by administering _____ .
    a. antihistamines
    b. epinephrine
    c. oxygen
    d. sublingual nitroglycerin

22. An allergic reaction involving the skin _____ .
    a. can develop into a life-threatening systemic reaction
    b. causes hives, wheals, a rash, and itching
    c. is treated with antihistamines
    d. A, B, and C

23. In an adult, systolic pressure of less than _____ is considered to be normal.
    a. 85
    b. 130

24. When the patient has been in a supine position for 2 or more hours, _____ may occur.
    a. hypoglycemia
    b. postural hypertension
    c. postural hypotension
    d. syncope

25. During a seizure, it is important _____ .
    a. not to place anything in the patient's mouth
    b. to firmly grasp the patient's tongue
    c. to place a padded tongue blade between the patient's teeth
    d. A or C

Competency 9 - 1 *Providing Emergency Treatment of Syncope*

Performance Objective: The student will demonstrate emergency care for a patient in a state of syncope in the dental chair. The patient is breathing and has no visible sign of injury of distress.

Important: *This will be performed in a treatment room with another student playing the role of the patient. A first aid kit, ammonia ampules, and gauze sponges should be available.*

Evaluator #1 (Name/date) _____

Evaluator #2 (Name/date) _____

Evaluator #3 (Name/date) _____

Check box if step was performed correctly.	1st	2nd	3rd
1. Asked patient, "Are you all right?" The patient did not respond.	☐	☐	☐
2. Called for help without alarming other patients.	☐	☐	☐
3. Placed patient in supine position with head slightly lower than his feet.	☐	☐	☐
4. Placed an ammonia ampule in a gauze sponge, then crushed the ampule.	☐	☐	☐
5. Wafted the ampule near, but not directly under, the patient's nose.	☐	☐	☐
6. Reassured patient as he regained consciousness.	☐	☐	☐

Notes:

Competency 9 - 2 *Taking and Recording Blood Pressure*

Performance Objective: The student will demonstrate taking and recording a patient's blood pressure.

Important: *A sphygmomanometer and a stethoscope are required for this procedure.*

Evaluator #1 (Name/date) _____

Evaluator #2 (Name/date) _____

Evaluator #3 (Name/date) _____

Check box if step was performed correctly.	1st	2nd	3rd
1. Gathered appropriate supplies.	☐	☐	☐
2. Explained procedure to the patient.	☐	☐	☐
3. Placed blood pressure cuff appropriately on the patient's arm.	☐	☐	☐
4. Placed stethoscope correctly in his or her ears.	☐	☐	☐
5. Placed the diaphragm of the stethoscope just above the elbow on the patient's brachial artery.	☐	☐	☐
6. Inflated the cuff and obtained systolic pressure reading.	☐	☐	☐
7. Deflated the cuff slowly and obtained diastolic pressure reading.	☐	☐	☐
8. Removed cuff and recorded readings.	☐	☐	☐
9. Prepared equipment for return to storage.	☐	☐	☐

Notes:

Competency 12 - 1 *Cleaning Up a Simulated Infectious Materials Spill*

Performance Objective: The student will use the appropriate exposure control methods to clean up a simulated spill of potentially infectious liquid on a hard surface floor.

Important: *Study both sides of this sheet before continuing.*

Evaluator #1 (Name/date) _____

Evaluator #2 (Name/date) _____

Evaluator #3 (Name/date) _____

Check box if step was performed correctly.	1st	2nd	3rd
1. Gathered appropriate supplies.	☐	☐	☐
2. Washed hands, put on utility gloves and other appropriate PPEs.	☐	☐	☐
3. Wet the area with a suitable disinfectant.	☐	☐	☐
4. Used a large wad of paper towels to wipe up area.	☐	☐	☐
5. Did not allow gloves to touch liquid and discarded towels appropriately after use.	☐	☐	☐
6. Applied disinfectant again and stated how long the area should be left wet.	☐	☐	☐
7. Dried the area with fresh paper towels and discarded the towels appropriately.	☐	☐	☐
8. Removed gloves without touching contaminated outside.	☐	☐	☐
9. Washed hands immediately and stated how utility gloves should be prepared for reuse.	☐	☐	☐
10. Followed the appropriate exposure control measures throughout the procedure.	☐	☐	☐

Notes:

Competency12 - 1 Instrumentation

Circle the appropriate icons if these
items would be used in actual patient
care.

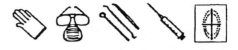

*List below all instruments, materials and supplies required for this
procedure.*

_____   _____

_____   _____

_____   _____

_____   _____

_____   _____

_____   _____

_____   _____

_____   _____

_____   _____

_____   _____

_____   _____

58

Competency 13 - 1 *Handwashing Before Gloving*

Performance Objective: Given the appropriate setting and equipment, the student will demonstrate handwashing before gloving.

Important: *A sink and handwashing supplies are required for this procedure.*

Evaluator #1 (Name/date) _____

Evaluator #2 (Name/date) _____

Evaluator #3 (Name/date) _____

Check box if step was performed correctly.	1st	2nd	3rd
1. Gathered appropriate supplies.	☐	☐	☐
2. Before gloving, removed all jewelry, including watch and rings.	☐	☐	☐
3. Regulated flow so the water was warm.	☐	☐	☐
4. Dispensed liquid soap and scrubbed hands vigorously.	☐	☐	☐
5. Rinsed, then scrubbed again.	☐	☐	☐
6. Worked soap under fingernails. If beginning of day, used orangewood stick and nail brush.	☐	☐	☐
7. Rinsed hands with cool water.	☐	☐	☐
8. Used a paper towel to dry hands and then forearms.	☐	☐	☐
9. If necessary, used towel to turn off water.	☐	☐	☐
10. Followed the appropriate exposure control measures throughout the procedure.	☐	☐	☐

Notes:

Competency 13 - 2 *Cleaning a Treatment Room After Patient Care.*

Performance Objective: The student will discard waste appropriately and use the "spray-wipe-spray" method to clean soiled surfaces in a treatment room. (The tray of soiled instruments has already been returned to the sterilization center.)

Important: *Study both sides of this sheet before continuing.*

Evaluator #1 (Name/date) _____

Evaluator #2 (Name/date) _____

Evaluator #3 (Name/date) _____

Check box if step was performed correctly.	1st	2nd	3rd
1. Gathered appropriate supplies.	☐	☐	☐
2. Washed hands and put on appropriate PPE.	☐	☐	☐
3. Removed soiled barriers.	☐	☐	☐
4. Sprayed soiled surface with a cleaning solution.	☐	☐	☐
5. Vigorously wiped surface after spraying.	☐	☐	☐
6. Sprayed surface with a disinfecting solution.	☐	☐	☐
7. Repeated steps 4, 5, and 6 until all soiled surfaces had been cleaned and disinfected.	☐	☐	☐
8. Discarded waste appropriately.	☐	☐	☐
9. Removed PPE and washed hands.	☐	☐	☐
10. Followed the appropriate exposure control measures throughout the procedure.	☐	☐	☐

Notes:

Competency 13 - 2 and 13 - 3 Instrumentation

Circle the appropriate icons if these items would be used in actual patient care.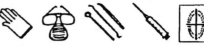

List below all instruments, materials, and supplies required for both of these procedures.

_____ _____

_____ _____

_____ _____

_____ _____

_____ _____

_____ _____

_____ _____

_____ _____

_____ _____

_____ _____

Competency 13 - 3 *Preparing a Treatment Room for Patient Care*

Performance Objective: The student will complete all of the steps required in preparing the treatment room prior to seating the patient.

Important: *Review the previous instrument list before proceeding.*

Evaluator #1 (Name/date) _____

Evaluator #2 (Name/date) _____

Evaluator #3 (Name/date) _____

Check box if step was performed correctly.	1st	2nd	3rd
1. Gathered appropriate supplies.	☐	☐	☐
2. Placed clean barriers.	☐	☐	☐
3. Prepared the patient's chart, radiographs, and laboratory work.	☐	☐	☐
4. Determined that the treatment room was ready with the dental chair in the proper position.	☐	☐	☐
5. Determined that all hoses and cords were out of the patient's way.	☐	☐	☐
6. Placed sterile instrument tray for next patient.	☐	☐	☐
7. Followed the appropriate exposure control measures throughout the procedure.	☐	☐	☐

Notes:

Competency 13 - 4 *Preparing Instruments for Recirculation*

Performance Objective: Provided with a tray of soiled instruments and the appropriate sterilization center equipment, the student will clean, wrap, sterilize (by autoclaving), and reassemble the contents of the instrument tray.

Important: *Study both sides of this sheet before continuing.*

Evaluator #1 (Name/date) _____

Evaluator #2 (Name/date) _____

Evaluator #3 (Name/date) _____

Check box if step was performed correctly.	1st	2nd	3rd
1. Gathered appropriate supplies.	☐	☐	☐
2. Washed hands and put on appropriate PPE.	☐	☐	☐
3. Discarded waste appropriately.	☐	☐	☐
4. Placed instruments in carrier, rinsed, and then ran through ultrasonic cycle.	☐	☐	☐
5. Rinsed instruments, removed from carrier, and placed on towel to dry.	☐	☐	☐
6. Bagged and sealed instruments for autoclaving.	☐	☐	☐
7. Either ran autoclave, or simulated same. Stated the time, pressure, and temperature required.	☐	☐	☐
8. Disinfected tray, removed PPE, and washed hands.	☐	☐	☐
9. Removed cool sterile instruments from autoclave and reassembled tray with all appropriate supplies.	☐	☐	☐
10. Followed the appropriate exposure control measures throughout the procedure.	☐	☐	☐

Notes:

Competency 13 - 4 Instrumentation

Circle the appropriate icons if these items would be used in actual patient care.

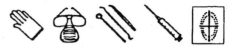

List below all instruments, materials, and supplies required for this procedure. Instruments are to be sterilized by autoclaving.

_____   _____

_____   _____

_____   _____

_____   _____

_____   _____

_____   _____

_____   _____

_____   _____

_____   _____

_____   _____

_____   _____

_____   _____

Chapter 14:
Dental Treatment Areas

Student's Name _____

Learning Objectives

Upon completion of this chapter, the student should be able to:

❑   Identify and state the use of each major piece of equipment in the dental treatment room.

❑   Describe or demonstrate the care and maintenance of each piece of dental equipment in the treatment room and laboratory.

❑   Demonstrate positioning the operator and assistant for rear, side, and front delivery of care.

❑   Identify and state the use of each major piece of equipment in the dental laboratory.

❑   Describe or demonstrate the morning and evening treatment room routine for the assistant.

❑   Demonstrate admitting, seating, and dismissal of the patient.

Exercises

Circle the letter next to the correct answer.

1.   When seated properly, the patient's _____ is/are fully supported.
     a.   buttocks
     b.   knees
     c.   lumbar region of the back
     d.   A, B, and C

2.   In preparation for seating the patient in the dental chair, the _____ .
     a.   arm on the entrance side is raised
     b.   chair is in the supine position
     c.   headrest is removed
     d.   A, B, and C

3. Before adjusting the operating light, it is first positioned _____ and then slowly adjusted upward.
   a. 15 to 25 inches below the patient's chin
   b. 25 to 30 inches below the patient's chin
   c. at the patient's chin
   d. at the patient's neck

4. The dentist's stool _____ have a ring near the base to support the feet.
   a. does
   b. does not

5. When the bulb of the operating light must be changed, this is done _____ .
   a. after the bulb has cooled
   b. after the patient has been dismissed
   c. as quickly as possible
   d. at the end of the day

6. Class _____ motions involve fingers-only movements.
   a. I
   b. II
   c. III

7. After the patient visit, the plastic saliva ejector is _____ .
   a. discarded
   b. disinfected
   c. sterilized

8. When cleaning the HVE system, the assistant's PPE includes wearing goggles and _____ .
   a. a face shield
   b. examination gloves
   c. utility gloves
   d. A and B

9. The dental chair is adjusted _____ the assistant puts on clean examination gloves.
   a. after
   b. before

10. In the _____ position, the patient's head and knees are on approximately the same plane.
    a. supine
    b. subsupine
    c. upright

11. The operator is seated with the thighs _____ .
    a. angled so that the knees are slightly above hip level
    b. angled so that the knees are slightly below hip level
    c. parallel to the floor

12. For use in cleaning the interior of the oral evaluation hoses, household bleach is mixed _____ of bleach to 2 quarts of water.
    a. 1 ounce
    b. 5 ounces
    c. 7 ounces
    d. 10 ounces

13. The adjustable curved bar from the back of the assistant's stool is positioned _____ .
    a. just below the assistant's rib cage
    b. to support the assistant when leaning forward
    c. to support the lumbar region of the back
    d. A and B

14. With _____ delivery, the dental unit is positioned to come over the patient's chest.
    a. front
    b. left-handed
    c. mobile

15. The properly seated dental assistant should _____ .
    a. be 4 to 5 inches higher than the operator
    b. be out of the operator's line of vision
    c. have his or her feet firmly supported
    d. A, B, and C

16. Attachments for the high- and low-speed handpieces are included on the _____ dental unit.
    a. assistant's
    b. operator's

17. The assistant's mobile cart is positioned _____ .
    a. at the assistant's side
    b. over the assistant's knees
    c. over the patient's chest

18. Extra supplies, such as gauze sponges, that are stored in a mobile cart must be _____ .
    a. disinfected prior to use
    b. packaged to maintain sterility

19. The model trimmer is used to _____ .
    a.   polish cast restorations
    b.   shape diagnostic casts
    c.   trim custom impression trays
    d.   A, B, and C

20. The central air compressor is used to supply compressed air to the _____ .
    a.   air-driven handpiece
    b.   air-water syringe
    c.   HVE tip
    d.   A and B

21. When changing the HVE and saliva ejector traps, it is necessary to _____ .
    a.   discard the used trap
    b.   handle the contaminated trap with tongs or cotton pliers
    c.   wear utility gloves
    d.   A, B, and C

22. The central vacuum provides the vacuum needed for the _____ .
    a.   air-water syringe
    b.   high-volume evacuator (HVE)
    c.   saliva ejector
    d.   B and C

23. The air-water syringe handle and hose are _____ .
    a.   classified as critical items
    b.   covered with a plastic barrier during the patient visit
    c.   must be sterilized after use
    d.   A and C

24. To prevent contamination, the curing light is _____ .
    a.   covered with a protective barrier before use
    b.   disinfected after use
    c.   sterilized after use
    d.   A and C

25. The uniform is worn _____ .
    a.   home if it is to be laundered
    b.   only in the office
    c.   to lunch if not using public transportation
    d.   A and C

72

Competency 14 - 1 *Identifying Treatment Room Equipment*

Performance Objective: The student will identify and state the purpose of each of the following major pieces of equipment in a dental treatment room: the dental chair, operating light, operator's stool, assistant's stool. The student will also be able to identify the dental unit(s) and carts, and the attachments included on each.

Important: *This procedure is to be performed in a dental treatment room. No additional instrumentation is required.*

Evaluator #1 (Name & date) _____

Evaluator #2 (Name & date) _____

Evaluator #3 (Name & date) _____

Check box if step was performed correctly.	1st	2nd	3rd
1. Demonstrated adjusting the height of the dental chair and placing it in the upright position.	☐	☐	☐
2. Demonstrated adjusting the operating light so it does not shine in the patient's eyes.	☐	☐	☐
3. Identified the operator's stool and the assistant's stool.	☐	☐	☐
4. Demonstrated the correct seated position of the assistant.	☐	☐	☐
5. Identified the assistant's unit or cart and identified the attachments on it.	☐	☐	☐
6. Identified the operator's unit or cart and identified the attachments on it.	☐	☐	☐
7. Identified the radiographic view box.	☐	☐	☐
8. Identified the curing light.	☐	☐	☐
9. Identified the amalgamator.	☐	☐	☐
10. Identified the sharps container.	☐	☐	☐

Notes:

Competency 14 - 2 *Seating and Positioning the Patient*

Performance Objective: The student will demonstrate seating the patient, placing the patient napkin, and placing the patient in the supine position.

Important: *A treatment room setting, a patient, a supply of patient towels, and a towel clip are required for this procedure.*

Evaluator #1 (Name & date) _____

Evaluator #2 (Name & date) _____

Evaluator #3 (Name & date) _____

Check box if step was performed correctly.	1st	2nd	3rd
1. Determined that the appropriate barriers were in place in the treatment room.	☐	☐	☐
2. Determined that the dental chair was in the proper position and other equipment out of the way.	☐	☐	☐
3. Determined that the patient chart, radiographs, and laboratory work were in place.	☐	☐	☐
4. Determined that the appropriate tray was in place.	☐	☐	☐
5. Escorted the patient to the treatment room.	☐	☐	☐
6. Seated the patient, placed personal objects (such as a handbag or glasses) in a safe place.	☐	☐	☐
7. If patient is female, asked her to remove lipstick.	☐	☐	☐
8. Cautioned patient before adjusting the chair position.	☐	☐	☐
9. Positioned chair so that the patient was in a supine position.	☐	☐	☐
10. Maintained patient comfort throughout.	☐	☐	☐

Notes:

Competency 15 - 1 *Identifying Dental Hand Instruments*

Performance Objective: Given an assortment of dental hand instruments, the student will identify each type of instrument. (The instructor may choose to give bonus points for correct identification of the primary use of each instrument.)

Important: *The instructor will prepare assorted hand instruments to be identified by numbering them from 1 through 10.*

Evaluator #1 (Name/date) _____

Evaluator #2 (Name/date) _____

Evaluator #3 (Name/date) _____

Check box if step was performed correctly.	1st	2nd	3rd
1. Correctly identified instrument #1.	☐	☐	☐
2. Correctly identified instrument #2.	☐	☐	☐
3. Correctly identified instrument #3.	☐	☐	☐
4. Correctly identified instrument #4.	☐	☐	☐
5. Correctly identified instrument #5.	☐	☐	☐
6. Correctly identified instrument #6.	☐	☐	☐
7. Correctly identified instrument #7.	☐	☐	☐
8. Correctly identified instrument #8.	☐	☐	☐
9. Correctly identified instrument #9.	☐	☐	☐
10. Correctly identified instrument #10.	☐	☐	☐

Notes:

Competency 15 - 2 *Identifying Dental Handpieces and Burs*

Performance Objective: The student will identify types of handpieces and burs (by shape). (The instructor may choose to give bonus points for correct identification of the number series for each type of bur.)

Important: *The instructor will prepare three handpieces (numbered 1 through 3) and seven basic burs (numbered 4 through 10).*

Evaluator #1 (Name/date) _____

Evaluator #2 (Name/date) _____

Evaluator #3 (Name/date) _____

Check box if step was performed correctly.	1st	2nd	3rd
1. Identified the type of handpiece #1.	☐	☐	☐
2. Identified the type of handpiece #2.	☐	☐	☐
3. Identified the type of handpiece #3.	☐	☐	☐
4. Identified the shape of bur #4.	☐	☐	☐
5. Identified the shape of bur #5.	☐	☐	☐
6. Identified the shape of bur #6.	☐	☐	☐
7. Identified the shape of bur #7.	☐	☐	☐
8. Identified the shape of bur #8.	☐	☐	☐
9. Identified the shape of bur #9.	☐	☐	☐
10. Identified the shape of bur #10.	☐	☐	☐

Notes:

Competency 16 - 1 *Positioning the HVE Tip*

Performance Objective: In a simulation, the student will demonstrate HVE tip placement for each area of the mouth

Important: *Required for this procedure are: a patient or manikin, a dental chair, a sterile HVE tip, sterile cotton rolls, and a sterile mouth mirror. Appropriate PPE is also required. It is desirable to have someone play the role of the operator.*

Evaluator #1 (Name/date) _____

Evaluator #2 (Name/date) _____

Evaluator #3 (Name/date) _____

Check box if step was performed correctly.	1st	2nd	3rd
1. Gathered appropriate supplies.	☐	☐	☐
2. Positioned HVE tip appropriately for maxillary right quadrant.	☐	☐	☐
3. Positioned HVE tip appropriately for maxillary left quadrant.	☐	☐	☐
4. Positioned HVE tip appropriately for maxillary anterior area.	☐	☐	☐
5. Positioned HVE tip appropriately for mandibular right quadrant.	☐	☐	☐
6. Positioned HVE tip appropriately for mandibular left quadrant.	☐	☐	☐
7. Positioned HVE tip appropriately for mandibular anterior area.	☐	☐	☐
8. Followed the appropriate exposure control measures throughout the procedure.	☐	☐	☐

Notes:

Competency 16 - 2 *Exchanging Dental Instruments*

Performance Objective: The student will demonstrate the exchange of dental instruments in a safe and efficient manner with the working end delivered in the position of use.

Important: *The instruments to be exchanged are determined by the instructor including examples of pen and palm grasp instruments. The instruments should be numbered from 1 through 10.*

Evaluator #1 (Name/date) _____

Evaluator #2 (Name/date) _____

Evaluator #3 (Name/date) _____

Check box if step was performed correctly.	1st	2nd	3rd
1. Passed instrument #1 in an acceptable manner.	☐	☐	☐
2. Passed instrument #2 in an acceptable manner.	☐	☐	☐
3. Passed instrument #3 in an acceptable manner.	☐	☐	☐
4. Passed instrument #4 in an acceptable manner.	☐	☐	☐
5. Passed instrument #5 in an acceptable manner.	☐	☐	☐
6. Passed instrument #6 in an acceptable manner.	☐	☐	☐
7. Passed instrument #7 in an acceptable manner.	☐	☐	☐
8. Passed instrument #8 in an acceptable manner.	☐	☐	☐
9. Passed instrument #9 in an acceptable manner.	☐	☐	☐
10. Passed instrument #10 in an acceptable manner.	☐	☐	☐
11. Followed the appropriate exposure control measures throughout the procedure.	☐	☐	☐

Notes:

Chapter 17:
Dental Radiography

Student's Name _____

Learning Objectives

Upon completion of this chapter, the student should be able to:

❑   Explain the responsibilities of the dentist and assistant relating to dental radiography safety.

❑   Describe the properties of x-radiation, explain how cumulative effects damage the body tissues.

❑   Identify the radiation exposure control steps taken in the dental practice.

❑   Describe the components of a dental x-ray machine and tube head.

❑   State how film quality is influenced by time, milliamperage, and kilovoltage.

❑   Identify normal anatomic landmarks processing and exposure errors as viewed on radiographs.

❑   Demonstrate treatment room preparations before seating the patient for exposing radiographs.

❑   Demonstrate producing diagnostic quality radiographs using the paralleling technique and the appropriate film holding devices.

❑   Demonstrate processing, mounting, and evaluating radiographs.

Exercises

Circle the letter next to the correct answer.

1. Dental radiographs show _____ .
    a. abnormalities in hard tissues
    b. changes in supporting structures
    c. dental decay
    d. A, B, and C

2. On a radiograph, the _____ appears radiolucent.
    a. dentin
    b. enamel
    c. sinus
    d. A and C

3. One sievert (Sv) equals _____ .
   a. 1 coulomb per kilogram (Ckg)
   b. 1 gray (Gy)
   c. 1 roentgen equivalent man (rem)
   d. 100 radiation absorbed doses (rads)

4. Milliamperage (mA) controls the _____ of electrons produced.
   a. number
   b. penetrating ability
   c. speed
   d. A, B, and C

5. The purpose of the filter in the head of the unit is to remove _____ .
   a. heat
   b. long wavelength x-rays
   c. low-energy x-rays
   d. B and C

6. The time between the exposure to x-rays and the appearance of clinical symptoms of excessive radiation is the _____ period.
   a. cumulative
   b. dormant
   c. latent
   d. somatic

7. Adult periapical radiographs normally require the use of film size _____ .
   a. 0
   b. 1
   c. 2
   d. 3

8. The patient's exposure to radiation can be minimized with _____ .
   a. accurate exposure technique
   b. a lead apron and thyroid collar
   c. rectangular collimation
   d. A, B, and C

9. Film holding devices are required when using the _____ technique.
   a. bisecting the angle
   b. paralleling

10. When exposing radiographs, the operator should **never** _____ .
    a. hold a film in the patient's mouth
    b. stand closer than 6 feet unless behind a protective barrier
    c. work without gloves
    d. A, B, and C

11. The properties of x-rays include the ability to _____ .
    a. penetrate matter
    b. travel at the speed of light
    c. travel in straight lines
    d. A, B, and C

12. The image quality of a radiograph is influenced by the _____ .
    a. focal spot size
    b. movement of the patient or film
    c. object-film distance
    d. A, B, and C

13. When placing the x-ray film in the mouth, the embossed dot or "bump" is always placed _____ the PID.
    a. away from
    b. toward

14. Exposure time is measured in _____ .
    a. impulses
    b. minutes
    c. seconds

15. Dental x-ray film should be stored away from _____ .
    a. heat
    b. moisture
    c. scatter radiation
    d. A, B, and C

16. An adult bite-wing survey usually includes _____ radiographs.
    a. 2
    b. 3
    c. 4
    d. 6

17. During exposure when the x-ray beam does not entirely cover the film _____ results.
    a. blurring of detail
    b. cone cutting
    c. horizontal distortion
    d. overlapping

18. Excessive vertical angulation can result in _____ of the image.
    a. elongation
    b. foreshortening
    c. overlapping

19. During processing of x-ray film, the _____ solution removes the undeveloped crystals from the emulsion.
    a. developer
    b. fixer

20. Overlapping of interproximal contact surfaces is a result of _____ angulation of the PID.
    a. excessive vertical
    b. improper horizontal
    c. insufficient vertical
    d. none of the above

21. Restorative materials that appear radiopaque on a radiograph include _____ .
    a. amalgam
    b. composite
    c. gold
    d. A and C

22. To locate teeth and pathologic conditions in a buccolingual direction, _____ radiographs are used.
    a. bite-wing
    b. occlusal
    c. periapical

23. For children under the age of 5 years, film size _____ is commonly used.
    a. 0
    b. 1
    c. 2
    d. 5

24. A/An _____ radiograph provides a view of the entire maxilla and mandible on a single film.
    a. cephalometric
    b. occlusal
    c. panoramic
    d. transcranial

25. With a _____ imaging system, the image is transmitted to, and stored in, the computer.
    a. digital
    b. panoramic
    c. xeroradiography
    d. none of the above

Competency 17 - 1 *Exposing an Adult Radiographic Survey Using the Paralleling Technique*

Performance Objective: The student will use the paralleling technique to produce a complete diagnostic quality radiographic survey. The number and types of exposures in the series are o be specified by the instructor.

Note: This procedure will be performed on a radiographic-type mannikin.

Important: *Study both sides of this sheet before continuing.*

Evaluator #1 (Name/date) _____

Evaluator #2 (Name/date) _____

Evaluator #3 (Name/date) _____

Check box if step was performed correctly.	1st	2nd	3rd
1. Gathered and prepared appropriate supplies.	☐	☐	☐
2. Seated the patient, placed the lead apron and thyroid collar, and explained the procedure.	☐	☐	☐
3. Positioned the patient appropriately for each exposure.	☐	☐	☐
4. Adjusted control panel settings appropriately for each exposure.	☐	☐	☐
5. Positioned the film and PID appropriately for each exposure.	☐	☐	☐
6. Exposed the prescribed number and type of films.	☐	☐	☐
7. Followed the appropriate exposure control measures throughout the procedure.	☐	☐	☐
8. Transported the exposed films to processing area.	☐	☐	☐

Notes:

Procedures 17 - 1, 17 - 2, and 17 - 3 Instrumentation

Important: *List here equipment and supplies required for all three of these procedures.*

Circle the appropriate icons if these items would be used in actual patient care.

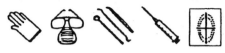

List below all instruments, materials, and supplies required for this procedure.

_____   _____

_____   _____

_____   _____

_____   _____

_____   _____

_____   _____

_____   _____

_____   _____

_____   _____

_____   _____

_____   _____

Competency 17 - 2 *Processing and Mounting Radiographs*

Performance Objective: The student will process and mount a series of dental radiographs that are free of processing errors.

Note: The instructor will indicate whether automatic or manual processing equipment is to be used.

Important: *Refer to the previous instrumentation list before proceeding.*

Evaluator #1 (Name/date) _____

Evaluator #2 (Name/date) _____

Evaluator #3 (Name/date) _____

Check box if step was performed correctly.	1st	2nd	3rd
1. Assembled supplies and prepared work area.	☐	☐	☐
2. Identified films with the patient's name and the date throughout processing and mounting.	☐	☐	☐
3. Processed exposed films appropriately for the method being used.	☐	☐	☐
4. Discarded contaminated film packets and lead foil in an appropriate manner.	☐	☐	☐
5. Films were free of processing errors.	☐	☐	☐
6. Left the processing area clean and ready for reuse.	☐	☐	☐
7. Placed identification on film mount.	☐	☐	☐
8. Placed radiographs in the appropriate windows of the radiographic mount.	☐	☐	☐
9. Followed the appropriate exposure control measures throughout the procedure.	☐	☐	☐

Notes:

Competency 17 - 3 *Evaluating Radiographs for Diagnostic Quality*

Performance Objective: The student will evaluate the series for diagnostic quality and determine the number of retakes required.

Important: *Review the previous instrumentation list before continuing.*

Evaluator #1 (Name/date) _____

Evaluator #2 (Name/date) _____

Evaluator #3 (Name/date) _____

Check box if step was performed correctly.	1st	2nd	3rd
1. Placed mounted survey on view box.	☐	☐	☐
2. Determined that the entire length of each tooth is visible and dimensionally accurate in at least one view.	☐	☐	☐
3. Determined that the apex of the roots of each tooth are visible in at least one view.	☐	☐	☐
4. Determined that 2 to 3 mm of surrounding tissues are visible in at least one view.	☐	☐	☐
5. Determined that each interproximal contact area is open in at least one view.	☐	☐	☐
6. Determined that contrast and density are adequate to show the details of the structures clearly.	☐	☐	☐
7. Identified number and position of retakes required.	☐	☐	☐
8. Stated the cause of each error and identified the action required to prevent a recurrence of that error.	☐	☐	☐

Notes:

Chapter 18:
Diagnosis and Treatment Planning

Student's Name _____

Learning Objectives

Upon completion of this chapter, the student should be able to:

❏   List and describe the three major steps in diagnosis and treatment.

❏   Discuss the assistant's role in diagnosis and treatment planning.

❏   List the eight areas of information covered during data gathering and describe the purpose of each.

❏   Describe the six clinical observations that are made regarding the patient's appearance.

❏   Identify types of cavities based on the cavity classifications as developed by G.V. Black.

❏   Identify the names and abbreviations used to describe the tooth surfaces involved in a cavity preparation or restoration.

❏   Demonstrate aiding a patient in completing a medical history form.

❏   Demonstrate recording the dentist's findings on a tooth diagram during an oral examination.

❏   Demonstrate recording scores on a PSR chart.

❏   Demonstrate recording patient treatment.

Exercises

Circle the letter next to the correct answer.

1. The patient's medical history is _____ .
   a. taken at the initial visit
   b. updated annually
   c. updated at each recall visit
   d. A and C

2. _____ is an examination technique in which the hands are used to feel the texture, location, and size of body parts.
   a. Bimanual manipulation
   b. Digital examination
   c. Palpation
   d. Palpitation

3. The patient's confidential medication history contains information concerning all _____ the patient is taking.
   a. illicit
   b. over-the-counter
   c. prescription
   d. A, B, and C

4. During the PSR examination, when the colored area of the probe completely disappears this is a score of _____ .
   a. 1
   b. 2
   c. 3
   d. 4

5. To examine hard-to-see soft tissue areas of the mouth, intraoral _____ is/are used.
   a. imaging on high magnification
   b. imaging on low magnification
   c. photographs
   d. radiographs

6. The cervical lymph nodes are examined for _____ .
   a. bruising
   b. swelling
   c. tenderness
   d. B and C

7. When the two halves of the face are not identical mirror images, the face is said to be _____ .
   a. asymmetrical
   b. disproportionate
   c. distorted
   d. symmetrical

8. To avoid triggering the gag reflex, the mouth mirror is _____ .
   a. cooled before placing it
   b. moved lightly across back of the tongue
   c. placed firmly on the back of the tongue
   d. A and C

96

Match the following cavity classifications and descriptions.

_____ 9. Class I cavities

_____ 10. Class II cavities

_____ 11. Class III cavities

_____ 12. Class IV cavities

_____ 13. Class V cavities

a. Abrasions involving the incisal edge or occlusal surface

b. Anterior interproximal

c. Anterior interproximal involving the incisal angle

d. Pit and fissure

e. Posterior interproximal

f. Smooth surface

14. To examine the tongue, a _____ is used to gently pull it forward.
    a. cotton pliers
    b. gauze sponge
    c. tongue retractor
    d. A or B

15. A compound cavity involves _____ surface(s) of the tooth.
    a. one
    b. two
    c. three or more

16. The abbreviation PFM stands for _____ .
    a. patient fainted momentarily
    b. porcelain filling on mesial
    c. porcelain fused to metal
    d. protrusive forward movement

17. The PSR _____ .
    a. does not replace a complete full mouth periodontal probing
    b. is particularly important for patients who have already been treated for periodontal disease
    c. is recommended for patients of all ages
    d. B and C

18. To palpate the _____, the fingers of each hand are gently placed just anterior to the tragus of each ear.
    a. carotid artery
    b. facial lymph nodes
    c. salivary glands
    d. temporomandibular joint

19. An appointment of _____ minutes is scheduled for the dentist to present the treatment plan to the patient.
    a. 5 to 10
    b. 10 to 15
    c. 15 to 20
    d. 30 to 45

20. When using a color-coding charting system, existing amalgam restorations are shaded in _____ .
    a. black
    b. blue
    c. green
    d. red

21. With a computerized charting system, a print-out of the examination findings is _____ .
    a. filed as part of the patient's chart
    b. given to the patient
    c. sent to the insurance company
    d. A and B

22. During the dental examination, the patient is placed in the _____ .
    a. position preferred by the operator
    b. subsupine position
    c. supine position
    d. upright position

23. To permit the operator visibility when examining under the tongue, the patient is instructed to _____ .
    a. move his tongue toward the cheek
    b. stick his tongue out
    c. touch his tongue to the hard palate
    d. A and C

24. For descriptive purposes during the PSR examination, the mouth is divided into _____ .
    a. quadrants
    b. sextants
    c. symmetrical halves

25. Of particular concern to the dentist are patient allergies to _____ .
    a. antibiotics
    b. latex
    c. local anesthetic solutions
    d. A, B, and C

98

Competency 18 - 1 *Obtaining Patient Health History Information*

Performance Objective: Given a health history form, the student will aid a "patient" (another student) in completing the form. (To protect privacy, the student serving as the patient can makeup a health history for this exercise.)

Important: *The instructor will provide the student with a health history form.*

Evaluator #1 (Name/date) _____

Evaluator #2 (Name/date) _____

Evaluator #3 (Name/date) _____

Check box if step was performed correctly.	1st	2nd	3rd
1. Explained to the patient the purpose of the form and emphasized the importance of answering all questions.	☐	☐	☐
2. Gave the patient the form and a pen or pencil.	☐	☐	☐
3. Gave the patient adequate time to complete the form.	☐	☐	☐
4. Reviewed the completed form to determine that all questions had been answered.	☐	☐	☐
5. Encouraged the patient to answer any remaining questions.	☐	☐	☐
6. If applicable, informed the dentist of any difficulties or questions regarding the questionnaire.	☐	☐	☐
7. Followed up on any "yes" or ambiguous answers.	☐	☐	☐
8. Thanked the patient for his or her cooperation.	☐	☐	☐

Notes:

Competency 18 - 2 *Recording a Dental Examination*

Performance Objective: Given a dental chart tooth diagram, the student will demonstrate recording the charting findings as dictated by the instructor.

Important: *The instructor will supply the student with a dental chart tooth diagram. The instructor will dictate an examination consisting of 10 items to be recorded on the diagram.*

Evaluator #1 (Name/date) _____

Evaluator #2 (Name/date) _____

Evaluator #3 (Name/date) _____

Check box if step was performed correctly.	1st	2nd	3rd
1. Recorded item #1 correctly.	☐	☐	☐
2. Recorded item #2 correctly.	☐	☐	☐
3. Recorded item #3 correctly.	☐	☐	☐
4. Recorded item #4 correctly.	☐	☐	☐
5. Recorded item #5 correctly.	☐	☐	☐
6. Recorded item #6 correctly.	☐	☐	☐
7. Recorded item #7 correctly.	☐	☐	☐
8. Recorded item #8 correctly.	☐	☐	☐
9. Recorded item #9 correctly.	☐	☐	☐
10. Recorded item #10 correctly.	☐	☐	☐

Notes:

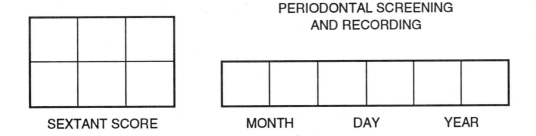

PERIODONTAL SCREENING AND RECORDING

SEXTANT SCORE   MONTH   DAY   YEAR

Competency 18 - 3 *Recording PSR scores*

Performance Objective: Using the diagram above, the student will record PSR scores by sextant as dictated by the instructor.

Important: *The instructor will dictate a score for each of the sextants.*

Evaluator #1 (Name/date) _____

Evaluator #2 (Name/date) _____

Evaluator #3 (Name/date) _____

Check box if step was performed correctly.	1st	2nd	3rd
1. Recorded sextant 1 correctly.	☐	☐	☐
2. Recorded sextant 2 correctly.	☐	☐	☐
3. Recorded sextant 3 correctly.	☐	☐	☐
4. Recorded sextant 4 correctly.	☐	☐	☐
5. Recorded sextant 5 correctly.	☐	☐	☐
6. Recorded sextant 6 correctly.	☐	☐	☐

Notes:

Date	Tooth	Service Rendered

Competency 18 - 4 *Recording Dental Treatment*

Performance Objective: Using the form shown above, the student will use the abbreviations taught in class to record treatment as dictated by the instructor.

Important: *The instructor should prepare a description of treatment that includes at least 5 items that must be included in the treatment record. This information is dictated to the students.*

Evaluator #1 (Name/date) _____

Evaluator #2 (Name/date) _____

Evaluator #3 (Name/date) _____

Check box if step was performed correctly.	1st	2nd	3rd
1. Recorded treatment item #1 correctly.	☐	☐	☐
2. Recorded treatment item #2 correctly.	☐	☐	☐
3. Recorded treatment item #3 correctly.	☐	☐	☐
4. Recorded treatment item #4 correctly.	☐	☐	☐
5. Recorded treatment item #5 correctly.	☐	☐	☐

Notes:

Chapter 19:
Alginate Impressions
and Diagnostic Casts

Student's Name _____ Marietta Pineda _____

Learning Objectives

Upon completion of this chapter, the student should be able to:

❑ List at least three uses of diagnostic casts.

❑ Discuss the differences between reversible and irreversible hydrocolloids and describe the two phases of all hydrocolloids.

❑ Explain why alginate impressions are not stored in water or exposed to the air.

❑ State the recommended water-powder ratios for model plaster, dental stone, and high-strength dental stone.

❑ List at least three factors that influence the setting time of gypsum products.

❑ Describe or demonstrate the procedure for obtaining a wax-bite registration.

❑ Demonstrate obtaining maxillary and mandibular alginate impressions.

❑ Demonstrate pouring, trimming, finishing, polishing, and labeling maxillary and mandibular diagnostic casts.

Exercises

Circle the letter next to the correct answer.

1. Diagnostic casts are used for _____ .
   a. creating athletic mouth guards
   b. fabricating orthodontic appliances
   c. treatment planning
   d. A, B, and C

2. When mixing a gypsum product, the warmer the water the _____ the set.
   a. faster
   b. slower

3. Normal-set alginate has a **working time** of _____ .
   a. 30 seconds
   b. 45 seconds
   c. 1 minute
   d. 2 minutes

4. Fast-set alginate has a **setting time** of _____ .
   a. 15 to 30 seconds
   b. 30 to 45 seconds
   c. 1 to 2 minutes
   d. 3 to 4 minutes

5. Alginate impression material is a/an _____ hydrocolloid.
   a. elastomeric
   b. irreversible
   c. reversible
   d. stable

6. The water-powder ratio for dental stone is 100 gm. of powder to _____ ml. of water.
   a. 20 to 25
   b. 30 to 32
   c. 45 to 50
   d. 50 to 75

7. When seating the mandibular impression tray, the _____ portion is pressed down over the teeth first.
   a. anterior
   b. lateral
   c. posterior
   d. either A or C

8. The water used for mixing alginate should be _____ ° F.
   a. 65 to 68
   b. 68 to 70
   c. 70 to 72
   d. 76 to 80

9. The impression tray selected must be deep enough to allow _____ mm of alginate between the tray and the incisal edges and occlusal surfaces of the teeth.
   a. 1 to 2
   b. 2 to 3
   c. 3 to 4
   d. none of the above

10. The art portion of the cast should be no more than _____ of the overall size.
    a. one-fourth
    b. one-third
    c. one-half

11. If stored in water, an alginate impression will _____ .
    a. absorb water
    b. change color
    c. dissolve
    d. shrink

12. Before being trimmed on the model trimmer, the casts should be _____ .
    a. cold and dry
    b. moist
    c. warm
    d. B and C

13. A metal impression tray that has been tried in the mouth but not selected, must be _____ .
    a. discarded
    b. disinfected prior to reuse
    c. immediately returned to storage
    d. sterilized prior to reuse

14. A mandibular alginate impression requires _____ scoops of powder and _____ measures of water.
    a. 2 / 2
    b. 2 / 3
    c. 3 / 3

15. Before impressions are handled in the laboratory, they must be _____ .
    a. autoclaved
    b. disinfected with a high-level disinfectant solution
    c. soaked in holding solution
    d. A and C

16. The anterior art portion of a maxillary cast is trimmed to _____ .
    a. a gently rounded curve
    b. an angle

17. If more water is added while mixing gypsum, the cast will _____ .
    a. be easier to pour
    b. be weaker
    c. set faster
    d. set slower

18. When taking alginate impressions of both arches, the _____ is usually taken first.
    a. bite registration
    b. mandibular impression
    c. maxillary impression

19. In the _____ method, the impression is surrounded with wax prior to pouring.
    a. box-and-pour
    b. double pour
    c. inverted-pour

20. Alginate is mixed with a _____ motion.
    a. brisk stirring
    b. fluffing
    c. spreading
    d. whipping

21. For a wax-bite registration, the patient is instructed to _____ .
    a. bite vigorously into the wax
    b. close normally
    c. make chewing motions
    d. A and C

22. When mixing a gypsum product, the _____ is placed in the bowl first.
    a. powder
    b. water

23. When using the model trimmer, the assistant must wear _____ .
    a. protective eyewear (as used during treatment)
    b. safety glasses
    c. utility gloves
    d. A and C

24. Alginate impression material deteriorates very quickly _____ .
    a. at elevated temperatures
    b. if stored in a lighted area
    c. in the presence of moisture
    d. A and C

25. Trimmed casts may be polished with a _____ .
    a. clean, dry cloth
    b. commercial gloss preparation
    c. soap and water solution
    d. A, B, or C

106

Competency 19 - 1 *Obtaining Alginate Impressions*

Performance Objective: The student will obtain diagnostic quality alginate impressions of the mandibular and maxillary arches.

Important: *Study both sides of this sheet before continuing.*

Evaluator #1 (Name/date) _____

Evaluator #2 (Name/date) _____

Evaluator #3 (Name/date) _____

Check box if step was performed correctly.	1st	2nd	3rd
1. Gathered appropriate supplies.	☐	☐	☐
2. Draped the seated patient and explained the procedure.	☐	☐	☐
3. Asked patient to take out any removable prosthesis.	☐	☐	☐
4. Used air-water syringe and HVE to rinse patient's mouth.	☐	☐	☐
5. Selected and modified the appropriate trays.	☐	☐	☐
Mandibular impression:			
6. Mixed impression material and loaded tray.	☐	☐	☐
7. Placed the loaded tray into patient's mouth and seated the tray properly.	☐	☐	☐
8. Removed tray when material was set. Used air-water syringe and HVE to rinse patient's mouth.	☐	☐	☐
Maxillary impression:			
9. Mixed impression material and loaded tray.	☐	☐	☐
10. Placed the loaded tray into patient's mouth and seated the tray properly	☐	☐	☐
11. Removed tray when material was set. Used air-water syringe and HVE to rinse patient's mouth.	☐	☐	☐
12. Rinsed and disinfected both impressions.	☐	☐	☐
13. Prepared supplies for disinfection or sterilization and return to storage.	☐	☐	☐
14. Followed the appropriate exposure control measures throughout the procedure.	☐	☐	☐

Notes:

Competency 19 - 1 and 19 - 3 Instrumentation

Important: *This list should include all materials and supplies for these three procedures.*

Circle the appropriate icons if these items would be used in actual patient care.

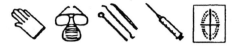

List below all instruments, materials, and supplies required for this procedure.

_____   _____

_____   _____

_____   _____

_____   _____

_____   _____

_____   _____

_____   _____

_____   _____

_____   _____

_____   _____

Competency 19 - 2 *Evaluating Mandibular and Maxillary Impressions*

Performance Objective: The student will evaluate the mandibular and maxillary impressions to determine that they are adequate to produce casts of diagnostic quality.

Important: *No supplies are required for this procedure.*

Evaluator #1 (Name/date) _____

Evaluator #2 (Name/date) _____

Evaluator #3 (Name/date) _____

Check box if step was performed correctly.	1st	2nd	3rd
Evaluating the mandibular impression:			
1. The impression shows that the tray was centered in patient's mouth.	☐	☐	☐
2. In critical areas, the impression material was smooth and free of voids.	☐	☐	☐
3. The retromolar pad was recorded in the impression.	☐	☐	☐
4. The peripheral roll was adequate.	☐	☐	☐
5. Each frenum was represented.	☐	☐	☐
6. The impression was acceptable.	☐	☐	☐
Evaluating the maxillary impression:			
7. The impression shows that the tray was centered in the patient's mouth.	☐	☐	☐
8. In critical areas, the impression material was smooth and free of voids.	☐	☐	☐
9. The tuberosity was recorded in the impression.	☐	☐	☐
10. The peripheral roll was adequate.	☐	☐	☐
11. Each frenum was represented.	☐	☐	☐
12. The impression was acceptable.	☐	☐	☐

Notes:

Competency 19 - 3 *Obtaining a Wax-Bite Registration*

Performance Objective: The student will obtain an acceptable wax bite registration. This procedure will be performed with a minimum of patient discomfort.

Important: *Supplies for this procedure are included on the previous instrumentation list.*

Evaluator #1 (Name/date) _____

Evaluator #2 (Name/date) _____

Evaluator #3 (Name/date) _____

Check box if step was performed correctly.	1st	2nd	3rd
1. Gathered appropriate supplies.	☐	☐	☐
2. Provided appropriate patient instruction.	☐	☐	☐
3. Prepared material appropriately.	☐	☐	☐
4. Placed softened wax on occlusal surfaces of the mandibular teeth.	☐	☐	☐
5. Instructed patient to close his teeth into the wax.	☐	☐	☐
6. Instructed patient to open his mouth and removed wax.	☐	☐	☐
Evaluated bite registration for adequacy			
7. Patient did not bite through wax.	☐	☐	☐
8. Patient bit hard enough to record occlusal surfaces.	☐	☐	☐
9. Bite registration was acceptable.	☐	☐	☐
10. Followed appropriate exposure control measures throughout the procedure	☐	☐	☐

Notes:

110

Procedure # 19 - 4 *Producing Diagnostic Casts in Plaster*

Performance Objective: The student will use the pouring procedure specified by the instructor to produce diagnostic casts in plaster. The wax bite will be used to articulate the casts as they are trimmed to an acceptable appearance.

Note: Criteria for acceptable appearance will be determined by the instructor.

Important: *Study both sides of this sheet before continuing.*

Evaluator #1 (Name/date) _____

Evaluator #2 (Name/date) _____

Evaluator #3 (Name/date) _____

Check box if step was performed correctly.	1st	2nd	3rd
1. Gathered appropriate supplies.	☐	☐	☐
2. Gently removed excess water from the impressions.	☐	☐	☐
3. Prepared a mix of plaster and poured each of the impressions.	☐	☐	☐
4. When the plaster had set, separated the impressions and cast without damage to the cast.	☐	☐	☐
5. Evaluated casts for diagnostic quality and determined that casts were free of voids in critical areas.	☐	☐	☐
6. Put on face shield or safety goggles, then used model trimmer to trim the casts to be esthetically acceptable.	☐	☐	☐
7. Placed patient identification on the casts.	☐	☐	☐
8. Left equipment and work area ready for reuse.	☐	☐	☐

Notes:

Procedure #19 - 4 Instrumentation

Circle the appropriate icons if these items would be used in actual patient care.

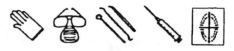

List below all instruments, materials, and supplies required for this procedure.

_____   _____

_____   _____

_____   _____

_____   _____

_____   _____

_____   _____

_____   _____

_____   _____

_____   _____

_____   _____

_____   _____

Chapter 20:
Pharmacology and Pain Control

Student's Name _____

Learning Objectives

Upon completion of this chapter, the student should be able to:

❏ Identify, by schedule, the major drugs covered by the Controlled Substance Act.

❏ Identify the major routes of drug administration and describe the procedures to be followed when handling medications.

❏ Describe three types of drugs used in dentistry for the control of anxiety, and differentiate between mild, moderate, and strong analgesics, giving an example of each.

❏ Describe the specialized uses and potential side effects (in dentistry) of the antibiotics penicillin, tetracycline, and erythromycin.

❏ Describe the uses of vasoconstrictors, corticosteriods, and atropine sulfate.

❏ Describe obtaining local anesthesia by block and by infiltration injection techniques.

❏ Identify the four stages of general anesthesia and describe the agents most commonly used to produce general anesthesia.

❏ Identify the three planes of nitrous oxide sedation in dentistry and identify the steps to be taken if the patient moves into the wrong plane.

❏ Demonstrate the placement of topical anesthetic ointment prior to an injection of a local anesthetic solution on the maxillary and mandibular arches.

❏ Demonstrate the preparation of an aspirating local anesthetic syringe, the proper disposal of the used needle, and the care of the used syringe.

Exercises

Circle the letter next to the correct answer.

1. _____ names are controlled by business firms, have registered trademarks, and are always capitalized.
   a. Brand
   b. Generic
   c. Prescription
   d. Trade

2. The _____ the gauge of a local anesthetic needle, the thicker the needle.
   a. higher
   b. lower

3. The action of drugs together so that the combined effect is greater than the effect of either drug taken alone is known as _____ .
   a. a secondary effect
   b. antagonism
   c. a toxic dose
   d. potentiation

4. Combined with local anesthetic solution, _____ may cause a dangerous increase in heart rate and blood pressure.
   a. alcohol
   b. cocaine
   c. morphine
   d. penicillin

5. Local anesthetic with epinephrine _____ recommended for patients with a history of heart disease.
   a. is
   b. is not

6. In general anesthesia, Stage _____ is known as surgical anesthesia.
   a. 1
   b. 2
   c. 3
   d. 4

7. A/An _____ is administered to reduce patient fears and tension.
   a. analgesic
   b. antianxiety agent
   c. hypnotic
   d. sedative

8. The needle guard is removed _____ .
   a. after the syringe has been placed in the operator's hand
   b. by the operator just prior to the injection
   c. prior to passing the syringe
   d. when the syringe is prepared

9. A Schedule IV drug _____ .
   a. has accepted medical usefulness
   b. has a low abuse potential
   c. may be dispensed by a written or oral prescription
   d. A, B, and C

114

10. If administered during the last trimester of pregnancy, _____ may produce permanent discoloration of the developing teeth.
   a. cephalosporin
   b. erythromycin
   c. penicillin
   d. tetracycline

11. Nitrous oxide sedation _____ be administered by a qualified EFDA under the general supervision of a dentist.
   a. may
   b. may not

12. The _____ on the local anesthetic syringe makes it possible to aspirate to be certain the needle has not entered a blood vessel.
   a. barrel
   b. harpoon
   c. hub
   d. piston rod

13. To minimize the secretion of saliva and mucus during some dental procedures, _____ may be administered.
   a. atropine sulfate
   b. emerol
   c. enflurane
   d. epinephrine

14. A short-acting local anesthetic lasts less than _____ .
   a. 30 minutes
   b. 1 hour
   c. 2 hours

15. If the patient becomes nauseated during the administration of nitrous oxide sedation _____ .
   a. all gases are discontinued immediately
   b. the flow of nitrous oxide-oxygen is decreased
   c. the flow of nitrous oxide-oxygen is increased
   d. 100 percent oxygen is administered immediately

16. A dental assistant _____ "call in" in a prescription for a controlled substance.
   a. may
   b. may not

17. Paresthesia, or persistent anesthesia, may be caused by _____ .
   a. hemorrhage into or around the nerve sheath
   b. the use of contaminated anesthetic solution
   c. trauma to the nerve sheath
   d. A, B, and C

18. The pressurized tank of _____ gas is green.
    a. nitrous oxide
    b. oxygen

19. A large air bubble in a local anesthetic cartridge is a sign that the solution has _____.
    a. been contaminated
    b. been exposed to sunlight
    c. been frozen
    d. passed the expiration date

20. Narcotics for office use _____ be ordered through a local pharmacy by prescription.
    a. can
    b. cannot

21. Drug administration by placement under the tongue is known as the _____ route.
    a. oral
    b. parenteral
    c. subcutaneous
    d. sublingual

22. Examples of strong analgesic drugs include _____ .
    a. aspirin
    b. Demerol
    c. Percodan
    d. B and C

23. By injecting the anesthetic solution in the proximity of the nerve trunk, _____ anesthesia is achieved.
    a. block
    b. infiltration
    c. intraosseous
    d. periodontal ligament

24. The blood vessels are constricted (narrowed) by _____ .
    a. bacitracin
    b. epinephrine
    c. morphine sulfate
    d. secobarbital

25. Corticosteroids are used _____ .
    a. as vasoconstrictors
    b. as vasodilators
    c. for the relief of pain
    d. to reduce inflammation

116

Competency 20 - 1 *Applying Topical Anesthetic*

Performance Objective: The student will gather the necessary equipment and then demonstrate the application of a topical anesthetic ointment in preparation for the injection of local anesthetic solution for the maxillary left central incisor.

Note: *This is an entry-level skill. The student should learn how to apply topical anesthetic ointment for every injection of local anesthetic solution in the mouth.*

Important: *Study both sides of this sheet before continuing.*

Evaluator #1 (Name/date) _____

Evaluator #2 (Name/date) _____

Evaluator #3 (Name/date) _____

Check box if step was performed correctly.	1st	2nd	3rd
1. Gathered appropriate supplies.	☐	☐	☐
2. Explained procedure to patient.	☐	☐	☐
3. Placed an appropriate amount of topical anesthetic ointment on cotton-tipped applicator.	☐	☐	☐
4. Used a sterile gauze sponge to gently dry the correct injection site.	☐	☐	☐
5. Removed gauze sponge. Positioned the applicator with the ointment directly on the injection site.	☐	☐	☐
6. Removed applicator after time recommended by the ointment manufacturer.	☐	☐	☐
7. Checked the comfort of the patient until the operator was ready to begin the procedure.	☐	☐	☐
8. Followed the appropriate exposure control measures throughout the procedure.	☐	☐	☐

Notes:

Competency 20 - 1, 20 - 2, and 20 - 3 Instrumentation

Circle the appropriate icons if these items would be used in actual patient care.

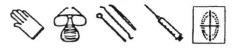

List below all instruments, materials, and supplies required for these procedures.

_____   _____

_____   _____

_____   _____

_____   _____

_____   _____

_____   _____

_____   _____

_____   _____

_____   _____

Competency 20 - 2 *Preparing a Local Anesthetic Syringe*

Performance Objective: The student will demonstrate the preparation of a local anesthetic syringe for an infiltration injection of anesthetic solution using an aspirating syringe and local anesthetic cartridge. The epinephrine ratio is specified by the dentist or instructor.

Important: *Use the instrumentation list from Procedure 20-1.*

Evaluator #1 (Name/date) _____

Evaluator #2 (Name/date) _____

Evaluator #3 (Name/date) _____

Check box if step was performed correctly.	1st	2nd	3rd
1. Gathered appropriate supplies.	❒	❒	❒
2. Disinfected needle end of anesthetic cartridge.	❒	❒	❒
3. Placed cartridge in syringe and engaged harpoon.	❒	❒	❒
4. Opened disposable needle packet without touching or contaminating the needle.	❒	❒	❒
5. Attached the needle to the syringe.	❒	❒	❒
6. Loosened the needle guard, but left it on the needle.	❒	❒	❒
7. Placed prepared syringe on the instrument tray out of the patient's sight.	❒	❒	❒
8. Followed the appropriate exposure control measures throughout the procedure.	❒	❒	❒

Notes:

Competency 20 - 3 *Caring for a Used Local Anesthetic Syringe*

Performance Objective: The student will demonstrate safely disassembling a used local anesthetic syringe in preparation for sterilization.

Important: *Reuse instrumentation list from Procedure 20-1.*

Evaluator #1 (Name/date) _____

Evaluator #2 (Name/date) _____

Evaluator #3 (Name/date) _____

Check box if step was performed correctly.	1st	2nd	3rd
1. Was still gloved from previous procedure.	☐	☐	☐
2. Recapped needle using a one-handed or needle holder technique.	☐	☐	☐
3. Removed needle and discarded appropriately.	☐	☐	☐
4. Removed the used anesthetic cartridge and discarded appropriately.	☐	☐	☐
5. Placed the syringe on the instrument tray to be returned to the sterilization center.	☐	☐	☐

Notes:

Chapter 21:
Coronal Polishing

Student's Name _____

Learning Objectives

Upon completion of this chapter, the student should be able to:

☐   Explain the difference between a prophylaxis and coronal polishing.

☐   State at least three indications and three contraindications for coronal polish.

☐   Name and describe five types of extrinsic stains found on the teeth.

☐   Describe the two categories of intrinsic stains found in the teeth.

☐   Name the tooth surfaces where a rubber cup is used, and those where a bristle brush is used.

☐   Describe the technique for using a prophy angle in terms of the grasp, handpiece speed, and positioning against the tooth.

☐   Describe at least four types of abrasives used in polishing teeth and state when each is used.

☐   Describe or demonstrate on each quadrant establishing a fulcrum or finger rest during coronal polishing.

☐   Describe or demonstrate proper operator and assistant seating for each quadrant during coronal polishing.

☐   In states where it is legal, demonstrate, on a typodont, coronal polishing technique.

Exercises

Circle the letter next to the correct answer.

1. During a coronal polishing procedure, the operator is seated with his or her
   _____ .
   a.   arms at waist level
   b.   back straight
   c.   feet flat on the floor
   d.   A, B, and C

2. Light stains on the tooth surface can be removed with _____ .
   a.   fine pumice
   b.   super-fine silex
   c.   zirconium

3. The coronal polishing procedure is indicated _____ .
   a. before a prophylaxis
   b. before dental dam placement
   c. to polish demineralized areas
   d. A, B, and C

4 The technique of polishing only those teeth with plaque or stain is called _____ .
   a. airbrasive technique
   b. generalized polishing
   c. incomplete technique
   d. selective polishing

5. Coronal polishing is not recommended for a patient with tuberculosis because the _____ .
   a. aerosol from the handpiece may spread the disease
   b. patient may have difficulty breathing
   c. procedure may cause bacteremia
   d. A and C

6. The prophy angle is held in a _____ grasp.
   a. palm
   b. palm-thumb
   c. pen

7. For coronal polishing, the recommended low-speed handpiece speed is _____ rpm.
   a. 10,000
   b. 20,000
   c. 100,000
   d. 200,000

8. Tetracycline is an example of a/an _____ stain.
   a. extrinsic
   b. intrinsic

9. A bristle brush should not be used on cementum or dentin because the surface is _____ .
   a. easily stained by the abrasive
   b. sensitive to the abrasive
   c. soft and easily grooved
   d. A and C

10. The use of fluoride prophylaxis paste _____ recommended before acid etching of enamel.
    a. is
    b. is not

11. Plaque and stain are removed from the interproximal areas with a/an
    _____ .
    a. abrasive
    b. dental floss
    c. rubber cup
    d. A and B

12. In preparation for a coronal polishing procedure, the patient should be
    covered with _____ .
    a. a patient towel
    b. a plastic drape
    c. protective eyewear
    d. A, B, and C

13. The _____ is/are are allowed to scale the teeth.
    a. dentist
    b. dental hygienist
    c. dental assistant
    d. A and B

14. To avoid injury to the gingival tissue, the rubber cup stroke should be
    directed _____ .
    a. away from the gingival tissue
    b. parallel to the gingival tissue
    c. toward the gingival tissue

15. When moving the rubber polishing cup from one area to another use a
    _____ motion.
    a. patting
    b. sweeping
    c. wiping
    d. A and C

16. The occlusal surfaces of the teeth are polished using a _____ .
    a. bristle brush
    b. rubber cup
    c. either A or B

17. To polish the buccal aspect surfaces of the maxillary left quadrant, the
    patient's head is turned _____ the operator.
    a. downward and away from
    b. downward and toward
    c. upward and away from
    d. upward and toward

123

18. When polishing the lingual aspect of the maxillary anterior sextant, the operator is seated at the _____ o'clock position.
    a. 6
    b. 8 to 9
    c. 10

19. The air-powder technique should not be used on a patient _____ .
    a. on a restricted sodium diet
    b. with a communicable disease that is spread by the handpiece aerosol
    c. with a respiratory disease
    d. A, B, and C

20. _____ is highly abrasive and is used only to clean highly stained teeth
    a. Chalk
    b. Course pumice
    c. Zirconium silicate

21. When performing a coronal polish, the left handed operator is usually seated at the _____ o'clock position.
    a. 3 to 4
    b. 8 to 9

22 Teeth that have been properly polished _____ .
    a. are glossy
    b. have a dull finish
    c. reflect light
    d. A and C

23 If using two polishing agents with different degrees of coarseness, the operator should use _____ .
    a. a separate rubber cup for each abrasive
    b. the finer abrasive on the rubber cup
    c. the coarser abrasive on the bristle brush
    d. B and C

24. When polishing the buccal aspect of the maxillary right posterior sextant _____ .
    a. establish a fulcrum on the maxillary right incisors
    b. have the patient tip his head up and slightly away from you
    c. hold the dental mirror in your left hand
    d. A, B, and C

25. The most common of the extrinsic stain found in children is _____ .
    a. black line
    b. green
    c. orange

Competency 21 - 1 *Coronal Polishing on a Typodont*

Performance Objective: The student will demonstrate coronal polishing technique on a typodont or mannikin.

Note: *In states where coronal polishing is legal, under proper supervision, the student will eventually perform this procedure on a patient. In other states, the student should be prepared to assist during a coronal polishing procedure.*

Important: *Study both sides of this sheet before continuing.*

Evaluator #1 (Name/date) _____

Evaluator #2 (Name/date) _____

Evaluator #3 (Name/date) _____

Check box if step was performed correctly.	1st	2nd	3rd
1. Gathered appropriate supplies.	☐	☐	☐
2. Positioned typodont correctly for each quadrant.	☐	☐	☐
3. Maintained correct operator position and posture for each quadrant.	☐	☐	☐
4. Demonstrated use of mouth mirror for retraction.	☐	☐	☐
5. Demonstrated use of mouth mirror for reflection of light.	☐	☐	☐
6. Maintained adequate fulcrum positions for each quadrant.	☐	☐	☐
7. Applied appropriate amount of polishing agent.	☐	☐	☐
8. Utilized a "pat and wipe" polishing stroke.	☐	☐	☐
9. Controlled handpiece speed and pressure throughout.	☐	☐	☐
10. Followed the appropriate exposure control measures throughout the procedure.	☐	☐	☐

Notes:

Competency 21 - 1 Instrumentation

Circle the appropriate icons if these items would be used in actual patient care.

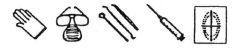

List below all instruments, materials, and supplies required for this procedure.

_____   _____

_____   _____

_____   _____

_____   _____

_____   _____

_____   _____

_____   _____

_____   _____

_____   _____

_____   _____

Competency 22 - 1 *Punching Dental Dam for Maxillary Anterior and Mandibular Posterior Placement*

Performance Objective: The student will demonstrate punching two dental dams, one for maxillary anterior placement and one the mandibular posterior placement.

Note: *The teeth to be exposed will be specified by the instructor.*

Important: *Study both sides of this sheet before continuing.*

Evaluator #1 (Name/date) _____

Evaluator #2 (Name/date) _____

Evaluator #3 (Name/date) _____

Check box if step was performed correctly.	1st	2nd	3rd
1. Gathered appropriate supplies.	☐	☐	☐
2. Marked specified holes for maxillary anterior placement.	☐	☐	☐
3. Punched holes for maxillary anterior placement.	☐	☐	☐
Evaluated maxillary dam preparation:			
4. Holes were appropriately sized.	☐	☐	☐
5. Holes were appropriately spaced and positioned.	☐	☐	☐
6. Holes were punched cleanly without ragged edges.	☐	☐	☐
7. Marked specified holes for mandibular posterior placement.	☐	☐	☐
8. Punched holes for mandibular posterior placement.	☐	☐	☐
Evaluated mandibular dam preparation:			
9. Holes were appropriately sized.	☐	☐	☐
10. Holes were appropriately spaced and positioned.	☐	☐	☐
11. Holes were punched cleanly without ragged edges.	☐	☐	☐
12. Followed the appropriate exposure control measures throughout the procedure.	☐	☐	☐

Notes:

Competency 22 - 1, 22 - 2, and 22 - 3 Instrumentation

Circle the appropriate icons if these items would be used in actual patient care.

List below all instruments, materials, and supplies required for the preparation, placement, and removal, of dental dam.

_____   _____

_____   _____

_____   _____

_____   _____

_____   _____

_____   _____

_____   _____

_____   _____

_____   _____

_____   _____

_____   _____

Competency 22 - 2 *Assisting in Dental Dam Placement*

Performance Objective: The student will assist the operator in the placement of the dental dam. (A mannikin may be used for this demonstration; however, appropriate exposure control protocols must be followed.)

Important: *Use the instruments listed on the previous instrumentation list.*

Evaluator #1 (Name/date) _____

Evaluator #2 (Name/date) _____

Evaluator #3 (Name/date) _____

Check box if step was performed correctly.	1st	2nd	3rd
1. Prepared appropriate supplies.	☐	☐	☐
2. Prepared clamp with a floss ligature.	☐	☐	☐
3. Placed clamp in dental dam forceps. Passed forceps to the operator in the position of use.	☐	☐	☐
4. Received clamp and forceps. Passed the clamp bow through the keyhole of the dam.	☐	☐	☐
5. Returned clamp, forceps, and dam to operator.	☐	☐	☐
6. Received forceps. Passed dental dam frame to the operator.	☐	☐	☐
7. Aided operator in passing dam between proximal contacts.	☐	☐	☐
8. Aided operator in inverting dental dam.	☐	☐	☐
9. Aided operator in ligating and stabilizing dental dam.	☐	☐	☐
10. Followed the appropriate exposure control measures throughout the procedure.	☐	☐	☐

Notes:

Competency 22 - 3 *Assisting in Removing Dental Dam*

Performance Objective: The student will demonstrate assisting the operator in the removal of dental dam. (A mannikin may be used for this demonstration; however, appropriate exposure control protocols must be followed.)

Important: *Use the instruments listed on the previous instrumentation list.*

Evaluator #1 (Name/date) _____

Evaluator #2 (Name/date) _____

Evaluator #3 (Name/date) _____

Check box if step was performed correctly.	1st	2nd	3rd
1. Had prepared appropriate supplies.	☐	☐	☐
2. Passed instrument to cut and remove ligatures.	☐	☐	☐
3. Received used instrument. Passed suture scissors to cut each dental dam septum.	☐	☐	☐
4. Received suture scissors. Passed dental dam clamp forceps.	☐	☐	☐
5. Received dental dam clamp forceps and clamp. Received dental dam frame and used dental dam.	☐	☐	☐
6. Checked dental dam for tears or missing pieces.	☐	☐	☐
7. Reported status of used dental dam to the operator.	☐	☐	☐
8. Used tissue to gently wipe patient's face clean.	☐	☐	☐
9. Used the air-water syringe and HVE tip to rinse the patient's mouth.	☐	☐	☐
10. Followed the appropriate exposure control measures throughout the procedure.	☐	☐	☐

Notes:

Student's Name _____ Marietta Pineda _____

Learning Objectives

Upon completion of this chapter, the student should be able to:

❏ List at least five factors that affect dental materials.

❏ Describe the steps in enamel bonding.

❏ Define smear layer and state why it is important in dentin bonding.

❏ List at least four types of dental cements and state the uses of each.

❏ Identify the important characteristics, uses, and means of manipulation of zinc phosphate, zinc oxide-eugenol, IRM, and glass ionomer cements.

❏ Describe the three types of fillers used in composite restorative materials and state when each is preferred. Also explain the differences between light-cured and self-cured composite restorative materials.

❏ Identify the major components of an amalgam alloy.

❏ Discuss the use and placement of cavity liners and bases.

❏ Demonstrate dispensing and mixing of the most commonly used dental cements either for luting a cast restoration or for use as a protective base.

Exercises

Circle the letter next to the correct answer.

1. Dental cements are used for _____ .
   a. fabricating diagnostic casts
   b. insulating bases
   c. permanent cementation
   d. B and C

2. Zinc oxide-eugenol cements _____ used under composite, glass ionomer, or other resin restorations.
   a. are
   b. are not

3. The ability of a liquid to flow is described in terms of its _____ .
   a. contact angle
   b. viscosity
   c. wetting ability
   d. A or C

4. A cavity liner is _____ a calcium hydroxide protective base.
   a. never placed with
   b. placed instead of
   c. placed over
   d. placed under

5. When placing cement into a crown, it is important to _____ .
   a. break up air bubbles that might have formed
   b. fill the crown entirely with cement
   c. ensure that the inner surfaces are covered
   d. A and C

6. In areas where strength is the primary concern, a/an _____ composite is used.
   a. hybrid
   b. macrofilled
   c. microfilled

7. Amalgam is condensed to _____ .
   a. aid in removing any excess mercury
   b. break up air bubbles in the mix
   c. compact the material tightly into the restoration
   d. A and C

8. Zinc phosphate cement is exothermic. This means that it _____ .
   a. absorbs water during mixing
   b. gives off heat during mixing
   c. gives off toxic fumes
   d. requires the use of a curing light

9. Glass ionomer cement is used as a _____ .
   a. bonding agent
   b. luting agent
   c. restorative material
   d. A, B, and C

10. When two metals touch in the mouth, a small shock is created. This is known as _____ .
    a. deformation
    b. galvanic action
    c. microleakage
    d. thermal conduction

11. The completed mix of polycarboxylate cement should be _____ .
    a. dull in appearance
    b. glossy
    c. stringy
    d. A and C

12. Before dentin bonding, the smear layer must be _____ .
    a. desiccated
    b. etched
    c. removed
    d. sealed

13. Bonding system materials _____ .
    a. can be used interchangeably
    b. consist of a liquid and a paste
    c. must be used according to the manufacturer's instructions
    d. A and C

14. A/An _____ restoration is expected to last about 6 months.
    a. amalgam
    b. intermediate
    c. permanent

15. Crushing pressure that pushes a material together is applied by _____ force.
    a. compression
    b. elastic
    c. shearing
    d. tensile

16. A/An _____ agent holds two things together.
    a. desiccating
    b. luting
    c. palliative
    d. A and B

17. A _____ cured composite is supplied as two pastes and polymerization occurs through a chemical reaction.
    a. light-
    b. self-

18. The slow release of fluoride in _____ cements inhibits recurrent decay.
    a. glass ionomer
    b. IRM
    c. zinc oxide-eugenol
    d. zinc phosphate

19. Copal cavity varnish is not compatible with _____ .
    a.   amalgam
    b.   composite restorative materials
    c.   glass ionomer cements
    d.   B and C

20. When working with light-cured composites, the darker the material the _____ the curing time.
    a.   longer
    b.   shorter

21. Immediately after it has been triturated, amalgam is _____ .
    a.   ready to be light-cured
    b.   soft and easily shaped
    c.   sticky and will adhere to the tooth
    d.   very strong

22. Zinc phosphate cement is mixed _____ .
    a.   on a paper pad
    b.   on a cool, thick glass slab
    c.   very quickly
    d.   B and C

23. Hardened zinc oxide-eugenol cement is removed from instruments by _____ .
    a.   soaking them in baking soda
    b.   wiping them with alcohol
    c.   wiping them with orange solvent
    d.   B or C

24. When IRM is supplied as a powder and liquid, it is mixed _____ .
    a.   on a glass slab
    b.   using a small flexible spatula
    c.   using a thick stiff flexible spatula
    d.   A and B

25. The setting reaction of glass ionomer cement is influenced by the _____ content of the liquid.
    a.   acid
    b.   activator
    c.   fluoroalminosilicate
    d.   water

Competency 23 - 1 *Mixing Zinc Phosphate Cement for Cementation*

Performance Objective: The student will assemble the necessary equipment and materials, then correctly manipulate the material for use in the cementation of a cast crown.

Note:. *If a crown is available, the student will also be asked to place the cement inside the crown.*

Important: *Study both sides of this sheet before continuing.*

Evaluator #1 (Name/date) _____

Evaluator #2 (Name/date) _____

Evaluator #3 (Name/date) _____

Check box if step was performed correctly.	1st	2nd	3rd
1. Gathered appropriate supplies.	☐	☐	☐
2. Read manufacturer's directions.	☐	☐	☐
3. Dispensed materials in the proper sequence and immediately recapped the containers.	☐	☐	☐
4. Incorporated powder into the liquid according to the manufacturer's directions.	☐	☐	☐
5. Completed the mix within the appropriate working time.	☐	☐	☐
6. Tested mass for droplet break 1 inch from slab.	☐	☐	☐
7. *Optional:* Filled the crown with cement.	☐	☐	☐
8. When finished, cleaned slab and spatula in preparation for sterilization.	☐	☐	☐
9. Returned supplies to storage or sterilization center.	☐	☐	☐
10. Followed the appropriate exposure control measures throughout the procedure.	☐	☐	☐

Notes:

Competency 23 - 1 Instrumentation

Brand of cement: _____

Circle the appropriate icons if these
items would be used in actual patient
care.

List below all instruments, materials, and supplies required for this
procedure.

_____   _____

_____   _____

_____   _____

_____   _____

_____   _____

_____   _____

_____   _____

_____   _____

_____   _____

_____   _____

Competency 23 - 2 *Mixing Zinc Oxide-Eugenol for a Sedative Base*

Performance Objective: The student will assemble the necessary equipment and materials, then correctly manipulate the material for use as a sedative base.

Important: *Study both sides of this sheet before continuing.*

Evaluator #1 (Name/date) _____

Evaluator #2 (Name/date) _____

Evaluator #3 (Name/date) _____

Check box if step was performed correctly.	1st	2nd	3rd
1. Gathered appropriate supplies.	☐	☐	☐
2. Read manufacturer's directions.	☐	☐	☐
3. Dispensed materials in appropriate amounts.	☐	☐	☐
4. Appropriately recapped containers immediately after use.	☐	☐	☐
5. Incorporated the powder and liquid according to the manufacturer's directions.	☐	☐	☐
6. Completed the mix to the proper thickness within the appropriate working time.	☐	☐	☐
7. When finished, cared for equipment in preparation for sterilization.	☐	☐	☐
8. Returned supplies to storage or sterilization center.	☐	☐	☐
9. Followed the appropriate exposure control measures throughout the procedure.	☐	☐	☐

Notes:

Competency 23 - 2 Instrumentation

Brand of cement: _____

Circle the appropriate icons if these
items would be used in actual patient
care.

*List below all instruments, materials, and supplies required for this
procedure.*

_____   _____

_____   _____

_____   _____

_____   _____

_____   _____

_____   _____

_____   _____

_____   _____

_____   _____

_____   _____

_____   _____

Student's Name _____

Learning Objectives

Upon completion of this chapter, the student should be able to:

❏ List the uses of custom trays and discuss the materials used to construct them.

❏ Differentiate between light-bodied, medium-bodied, and heavy-bodied elastomeric impression materials and state one use of each.

❏ Explain the purpose of the occlusal registration and describe the use of the triple tray technique to obtain this impression.

❏ Demonstrate the construction and finishing of a custom impression tray.

❏ Demonstrate the preparation of at least two types of elastomeric impression materials.

❏ Demonstrate assisting during the two-step impression technique using silicone impression materials.

Exercises

Circle the letter next to the correct answer.

1. The centric relationship of the upper and lower arches is obtained in the _____ registration.
    a. bite
    b. occlusal
    c. A and/or B

2. The impression tray is treated with a/an _____ to retain the elastomeric material within the tray.
    a. accelerator
    b. adhesive
    c. surfactant
    d. wetting agent

3. Custom trays are constructed using _____.
   a. alginate
   b. polysulfide
   c. self-curing acrylic resin
   d. B and C

4. Polysiloxane is a type of _____ silicone impression material.
   a. addition
   b. condensation

5. The vacuum former is used to create _____.
   a. impression trays
   b. mouth guards
   c. nightguard vital bleaching trays
   d. A, B, and C

6. In a/an _____ bite registration technique, the patient is instructed to bring his teeth together before the impression material is placed.
   a. closed
   b. open
   c. triple tray

7. Impression materials that do not react well to moisture are said to be _____.
   a. hydrophobic
   b. hydrophilic

8. Overgloves must be worn when handling _____ impression putty.
   a. addition silicone
   b. condensation silicone
   c. polysulfide

9. If _____ are present on the cast, they may make it impossible to properly seat or remove the custom tray.
   a. anatomic landmarks
   b. partially erupted teeth
   c. undercuts
   d. A and C

10. _____ impression materials have a very strong odor and will permanently stain clothing.
    a. Polyether
    b. Polysulfide
    c. Silicone
    d. A, B, and C

11. To prevent the custom tray from seating too far on the arch, _____ are created in the tray.
    a. spacers
    b. stops

12. Light-bodied impression material is also referred to as _____ .
    a. a wash
    b. putty type
    c. syringe type
    d. A and C

13. A thinner is used to reduce the thickness of the mix of _____ impression material.
    a. addition silicone
    b. polyether
    c. polysulfide
    d. none of the above

14. The reaction that changes elastomeric impression materials from a paste into a rubber-like material is called _____ .
    a. deformation
    b. manipulation
    c. polymerization

15. The handle of a custom tray is placed _____ .
    a. at the anterior
    b. facing out of the mouth
    c. near the midline
    d. A, B, and C

16. The extruder gun is loaded with dual cartridges, one each of _____ type material.
    a. catalyst and base
    b. polysulfide and silicone
    c. syringe and heavy-bodied
    d. wash and condensation putty

17. After use, the dispenser tip of an impression syringe or extruder gun is _____ .
    a. discarded
    b. disinfected
    c. sterilized

18. When accuracy is extremely important, an _____ impression material is used.
    a. alginate
    b. elastomeric

19. _____ impression materials are sometimes used in a two-step procedure with a preliminary impression taken before the teeth are prepared.
    a. Alginate
    b. Polyether
    c. Polysulfide
    d. Silicone

20. A self-curing acrylic resin tray may be removed from the cast after it reaches initial set in approximately _____ minutes.
    a. 3 to 4
    b. 5 to 6
    c. 7 to 10
    d. 10 to 15

21. The mixing time for condensation silicone impression materials is approximately _____ seconds.
    a. 30 to 45
    b. 30 to 60
    c. 60

22. A thermoplastic tray plastic is made workable by _____ .
    a. a chemical reaction
    b. heat
    c. placing it in the vacuum former

23. When completing a custom tray, the spacer is _____ .
    a. left in place and painted with adhesive
    b. melted away by the heat of the acrylic
    c. removed and the tray is cleaned

24. A/An _____ impression material must be used in a clear plastic tray.
    a. elastomeric
    b. hydrophilic
    c. light-cured
    d. putty

25. Before it is placed on the vacuum former, the cast must be _____ .
    a. thoroughly dry
    b. heated
    c. soaked in water
    d. A and B

146

Competency 24 - 1 *Constructing a Custom Impression Tray*

Performance Objective: The student will construct a full arch custom tray for a mandibular impression using acrylic resin tray material and wax spacing material.

Important: *Study both sides of this sheet before continuing.*

Evaluator #1 (Name/date) _____

Evaluator #2 (Name/date) _____

Evaluator #3 (Name/date) _____

Check box if step was performed correctly.	1st	2nd	3rd
1. Gathered the appropriate supplies.	☐	☐	☐
2. Evaluated the cast and eliminated defects that would impair placement or removal of the tray.	☐	☐	☐
3. Placed the spacer.	☐	☐	☐
4. Prepared the stops.	☐	☐	☐
5. Painted the spacer and surrounding area with separating medium.	☐	☐	☐
6. Mixed and placed the tray material.	☐	☐	☐
7. Prepared and placed the tray handle.	☐	☐	☐
8. After the initial set, removed the spacer and replaced the tray on the cast to complete the set.	☐	☐	☐

Evaluated the completed tray for acceptability

	1st	2nd	3rd
9. The tray covered the desired area.	☐	☐	☐
10. The stops were properly positioned.	☐	☐	☐
11. The handle was appropriately placed.	☐	☐	☐
12. Smoothed edges of tray as necessary.	☐	☐	☐
13. Painted interior of tray with the appropriate adhesive.	☐	☐	☐

Notes:

Competency 24 - 1 Instrumentation

Circle the appropriate icons if these items would be used in actual patient care.

List below all instruments, materials, and supplies required for this procedure.

_____   _____

_____   _____

_____   _____

_____   _____

_____   _____

_____   _____

_____   _____

_____   _____

_____   _____

_____   _____

_____   _____

148

Competency 24 - 2 Mixing Syringe-Type and Tray-Type Impression Materials

Performance Objective: The student will follow the manufacturer's instructions for mixing the impression materials selected by the instructor. The custom tray fabricated by the student may be used in this procedure.

Note: The instructor will select the type of impression materials to be mixed.

Important: *Study both sides of this sheet before continuing.*

Evaluator #1 (Name/date) _____

Evaluator #2 (Name/date) _____

Evaluator #3 (Name/date) _____

Check box if step was performed correctly.	1st	2nd	3rd
1. Gathered the appropriate supplies.	☐	☐	☐
2. Followed the manufacturer's directions for dispensing and mixing the syringe-type material.	☐	☐	☐
3. If applicable, loaded and passed the impression syringe.	☐	☐	☐
4. Followed the manufacturer's directions for dispensing and mixing the tray-type material.	☐	☐	☐
5. Loaded and passed the impression tray.	☐	☐	☐
6. Described how the completed impression would be disinfected.	☐	☐	☐
7. Prepared supplies and equipment to be returned to the sterilization center.	☐	☐	☐
8. Followed the appropriate exposure control measures throughout the procedure.	☐	☐	☐

Notes:

Competency 24 - 2 Instrumentation

Brand: _____

Circle the appropriate icons if these
items would be used in actual patient
care.

*List below all instruments, materials, and supplies required for this
procedure.*

_____   _____

_____   _____

_____   _____

_____   _____

_____   _____

_____   _____

_____   _____

_____   _____

_____   _____

_____   _____

Competency 24 - 3 *Assisting in a Two-Step Impression Technique*

Performance Objective: The student will prepare the impression materials and care for the impression during a two-step technique using silicone impression materials.

Note: A typodont will be used to simulate taking the preliminary impression.

Important: *Study both sides of this sheet before continuing.*

Evaluator #1 (Name/date) _____

Evaluator #2 (Name/date) _____

Evaluator #3 (Name/date) _____

Check box if step was performed correctly.	1st	2nd	3rd
1. Gathered the appropriate supplies including an impression tray painted with adhesive.	☐	☐	☐
2. Mixed putty base according to the manufacturer's directions.	☐	☐	☐
3. Loaded the putty into the impression tray.	☐	☐	☐
4. Placed an indentation in impression material where the teeth will be.	☐	☐	☐
5. Placed plastic sheet spacer over impression material.	☐	☐	☐
6. Passed the tray to the operator or placed the tray on the typodont.	☐	☐	☐
7. Removed the spacer from the impression and checked for defects (large bubbles or wrinkles).	☐	☐	☐
8. Used a scalpel to trim away undercuts in the impression.	☐	☐	☐
9. Cared for the impression appropriately until time to take the second impression.	☐	☐	☐
10. Described preparation of the extruder gun with wash and the steps in the final impression.	☐	☐	☐
11. Cared for the completed impression appropriately.	☐	☐	☐
12. Prepared supplies and equipment to be returned to the sterilization center.	☐	☐	☐
13. Followed the appropriate exposure control measures throughout the procedure.	☐	☐	☐

Notes:

Competency 24 - 3 Instrumentation

Brand: _____

Circle the appropriate icons if these
items would be used in actual patient
care.

*List below all instruments, materials, and supplies required for this
procedure.*

_____   _____

_____   _____

_____   _____

_____   _____

_____   _____

_____   _____

_____   _____

_____   _____

_____   _____

Chapter 25:
Restorative and Cosmetic Dentistry

Student's Name _____ Marietta Pineda _____

Learning Objectives

Upon completion of this chapter, the student should be able to:

☐   Define the terms cavity walls, line angles, point angles and describe the principles of cavity preparation.

☐   State the steps in bonding an amalgam restoration.

☐   Describe the placement of direct bonded composite veneers.

☐   Discuss the preparation, application, and removal of a matrix for a Class II amalgam restoration and for a Class II composite restoration.

☐   Describe the materials and the procedure for in-office and nightguard bleaching of vital teeth.

☐   Identify the instrumentation required for the placement of a Class III composite restoration and a Class II amalgam restoration.

☐   Demonstrate the role of a chairside assistant in the preparation and placement of a Class II amalgam restoration.

☐   Demonstrate the role of a chairside assistant in the preparation and placement of a Class III composite restoration.

Exercises

Circle the letter next to the correct answer.

1.   When placing a Class III restoration, a _____ matrix is used.
      a.   clear plastic strip
      b.   crown form
      c.   Tofflemire

2.   The junction of two walls in the cavity preparation form a _____ angle.
      a.   line
      b.   point

153

3. Amalgam is used as a restorative material because it _____ .
   a. forms a direct bond with the tooth structure
   b. is soft and easily shaped when freshly mixed
   c. provides the strength that is important in posterior restorations
   d. B and C

4. When condensing amalgam, the operator begins with the _____ condenser.
   a. largest
   b. smallest

5. Supervised nightguard bleaching _____ .
   a. is usually effective on teeth stained by coffee, tea, or smoking
   b. is recommended for nonvital teeth
   c. produces permanent results
   d. A, B, and C

6. When placing a Class I restoration, a matrix _____ required.
   a. is
   b. is not

7. Articulating paper will leave colored marks on _____ of a freshly placed restoration.
   a. high spots
   b. interproximal areas
   c. overhangs

8. The _Diagonal slot_ of the Tofflemire matrix retainer positions the band securely within the retainer.
   a. inner knob
   b. outer knob
   c. spindle

9. When placing a direct bonded composite veneer _____ .
   a. an opaquer may be used under the veneer to block out stains
   b. local anesthesia is required
   c. the shade is selected after the dental dam has been placed
   d. A, B, and C

10. The wedge is most commonly placed from the _____ side into the interproximal space.
    a. buccal
    b. facial
    c. lingual
    d. A or B

154

11. When placing a Class V composite restoration, the restorative material is
_____ .
   a. loaded into the contoured matrix and then forced into the preparation
   b. placed directly into the prepared tooth
   c. A or B

12. Amalgam bonding _____ mechanical retention.
   a. is supplemental to
   b. replaces

13. The slotted surface of the retainer is always positioned toward the _____ .
   a. facial surface
   b. gingiva
   c. incisal edge
   d. occlusal surface

14. _____ composites are mixed to achieve the correct shade.
   a. Light-cured
   b. Self-curing

Match the following terms and definitions.

___ 15.   Convenience form

___ 16.   Outline form

___ 17.   Resistance form

a. The curved shape and border of the restoration and enamel at the tooth surface

b. The shape and relationship of the cavity walls that protect the tooth structure and restorative material against fracture

c. The shape and relationship of the cavity walls that provide mechanical retention

d. The size of the cavity opening required to allow the operator access to the cavity preparation

18. With a retainerless matrix system, the used band is _____
    a. discarded with the sharps
    b. disinfected before reuse
    c. sterilized before reuse

19. When placing a Class I composite restoration, _____ .
    a. a eugenol-free cavity liner is placed
    b. a matrix band is not required
    c. nonstick plastic or highly polished stainless steel placement instruments are used
    d. A, B, and C

20. The walking bleach technique _____ .
    a. is performed by the patient at home
    b. is used only on nonvital teeth
    c. requires a custom tray
    d. A, B, and C

21. When placing a composite restoration, the tooth is etched _____ the matrix band is placed.
    a. after
    b. before

22. Retention pins are held in place by _____ .
    a. bonding
    b. the restorative material
    c. zinc phosphate cement

23. When placing a Class II amalgam restoration, the occlusal surface is carved _____ .
    a. after the matrix band has been removed
    b. after the restoration has been light-cured
    c. using an explorer
    d. using a high-speed handpiece

24. The used amalgam capsule is reassembled immediately to _____ .
    a. minimize mercury escaping into the air
    b. prepare the capsule for reuse
    c. save the extra amalgam for later use

25. When placing a matrix, an egg-shaped burnisher is used to _____ .
    a. contour the band
    b. seat the band on the tooth
    b. seat the wedge
    b. smooth and shape the occlusal edge of the band

Competency 25 - 1 *Assisting in the Placement of an Amalgam Restoration*

Performance Objective: The student will demonstrate the role of the chairside assistant throughout all steps in the preparation, placement, and finishing of a Class II amalgam restoration

Note: *The treatment area has been cleaned and protective barriers are in place. All supplies are in place and the patient has been seated and positioned. Local anesthetic has been administered. (The operator did not elect to use dental dam.)*

Important: *Study both sides of this sheet before continuing.*

Evaluator #1 (Name/date) _____

Evaluator #2 (Name/date) _____

Evaluator #3 (Name/date) _____

Check box if step was performed correctly.	1st	2nd	3rd
1. Anticipated operator's needs and demonstrated effective and appropriate use of the HVE and air-water syringe.	☐	☐	☐
2. Anticipated operator's needs and demonstrated effective and appropriate soft tissue retraction.	☐	☐	☐
3. Anticipated operator's needs and demonstrated effective and appropriate exchange of instruments and materials.	☐	☐	☐
4. Mixed and passed (or placed) cavity liner and base in appropriate quantity and sequence.	☐	☐	☐
5. Assembled, passed, or placed matrix band and wedge.	☐	☐	☐
6. Mixed amalgam and loaded amalgam carriers.	☐	☐	☐
7. Exchanged amalgam carriers and condensers as needed.	☐	☐	☐
8. Assisted in matrix removal and passed carving instruments.	☐	☐	☐
9. Passed (or placed) articulating paper and passed carvers as needed.	☐	☐	☐
10. Rinsed patient's mouth to remove debris and excess water.	☐	☐	☐
11. Anticipated operator needs throughout the procedure.	☐	☐	☐
12. Followed the appropriate exposure control measures throughout the procedure.	☐	☐	☐

Notes:

Competency 25 - 1 Instrumentation

Circle the appropriate icons if these items would be used in actual patient care.

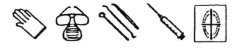

Although the instruments should already be in place for this procedure, the student should complete the instrumentation list so he or she will be able to determine whether or not any of the necessary supplies are missing.

_____ _____

_____ _____

_____ _____

_____ _____

_____ _____

_____ _____

_____ _____

_____ _____

_____ _____

_____ _____

158

Competency 25 - 2 *Assisting in the Placement of a Composite Restoration*

Performance Objective: The student will demonstrate the role of the chairside assistant throughout all steps in the preparation, placement, and finishing of a Class III light-cured composite restoration

Note: The treatment area has been cleaned and protective barriers are in place. All supplies are in place and the patient has been seated and positioned. No local anesthetic is required. (The operator did not elect to use dental dam.) No liner or base is required.

Important: *Study both sides of this sheet before continuing.*

Evaluator #1 (Name/date) _____

Evaluator #2 (Name/date) _____

Evaluator #3 (Name/date) _____

Check box if step was performed correctly.	1st	2nd	3rd
1. Anticipated operator's needs and demonstrated effective and appropriate use of the HVE and air-water syringe.	☐	☐	☐
2. Anticipated operator's needs and demonstrated effective and appropriate soft tissue retraction.	☐	☐	☐
3. Anticipated operator's needs and demonstrated effective and appropriate exchange of instruments and materials.	☐	☐	☐
4. Assisted in placement of the matrix.	☐	☐	☐
5. Anticipated and demonstrated appropriate help during the etching procedure and application of bonding agent.	☐	☐	☐
6. Passed composite of the appropriate shade.	☐	☐	☐
7. Passed or held the curing light as directed.	☐	☐	☐
8. Assisted in removing matrix.	☐	☐	☐
9. Prepared and passed handpiece and/or hand instruments for finishing restoration.	☐	☐	☐
10. Rinsed patient's mouth to remove debris and excess water.	☐	☐	☐
11. Anticipated operator needs throughout the procedure.	☐	☐	☐
12. Followed the appropriate exposure control measures throughout the procedure.	☐	☐	☐

Notes:

Competency 25 - 2 Instrumentation

Circle the appropriate icons if these items would be used in actual patient care.

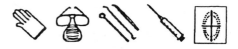

Although the instruments should already be in place for this procedure, the student should complete the instrumentation list so he or she will be able to determine whether or not any of the necessary supplies are missing.

_____   _____

_____   _____

_____   _____

_____   _____

_____   _____

_____   _____

_____   _____

_____   _____

_____   _____

_____   _____

Chapter 26: Periodontics

Student's Name _____

Learning Objectives

Upon completion of this chapter, the student should be able to:

❏   State the roles of the registered dental hygienist and dental assistant in periodontics.

❏   Describe the steps in a complete periodontal examination.

❏   Identify the specialized instruments used in periodontics.

❏   Describe these periodontal procedures: prophylaxis, scaling and curettage, root planing, gingivectomy, gingivoplasty, and osteoplasty.

❏   Discuss the points to be covered when giving postoperative instructions to a patient following periodontal surgery.

❏   Demonstrate preparing an instrument tray for periodontal surgery.

❏   Demonstrate mixing noneugenol periodontal surgical dressing.

Exercises

Circle the letter next to the correct answer.

1. A periodontal examination and diagnosis includes _____ .
   a. evaluation of radiographs
   b. medical and dental histories
   c. periodontal probing and recording
   d. A, B, and C

2. Calculus _____ be removed by brushing and other plaque control methods.
   a. can
   b. cannot

3. The primary cause of gingivitis and most forms of periodontal disease is _____ .
   a. calculus
   b. defective restorations
   c. food debris
   d. plaque

4. The depth of a periodontal pocket is measured with a/an _____ .
   a. curette
   b. explorer
   c. periodontal probe
   d. pocket marker

5. The _____ is/are licensed to perform a dental prophylaxis.
   a. dental assistant
   b. dentist
   c. registered dental hygienist
   d. B and C

6. A gingivectomy is indicated for the removal of _____ .
   a. gingival enlargements
   b. osseous defects
   c. suprabony periodontal abscesses
   d. A and C

7. To surgically reshape the bone to remove defects and to restore normal contours, a/an _____ is performed.
   a. curettage
   b. gingivoplasty
   c. osteoplasty
   d. root planing

8. An inflammatory process that occurs when the gingiva surrounding a partially erupted tooth becomes infected is known as _____ .
   a. acute necrotizing ulcerative gingivitis
   b. a periodontal abscess
   c. gingivitis
   d. pericoronitis

9. In periodontics, a laser may be used to _____ .
   a. control bleeding
   b. remove excess bone
   c. remove tumors and lesions
   d. A and C

10. Probing of periodontal pockets may legally be performed by the _____ .
    a. dentist and dental hygienist
    b. EFDA
    c. registered dental assistant
    d. A and B

11. During an examination, the bleeding index is based on the principle that
_____ .
  a.   bleeding during probing is an indication of a blood disorder
  b.   healthy gingiva does not bleed
  c.   it is normal for probing to cause moderate bleeding

12. Occlusal trauma causes _____ .
  a.   gingival hyperplasia
  b.   pocket formation
  c.   tooth mobility
  d.   A, B, and C

13. To locate calculus deposits, a/an _____ is used.
  a.   explorer
  b.   curette
  c.   periodontal probe

14. The procedure that removes calculus, soft deposits, and stain from all
unattached tooth surfaces is known as _____ .
  a.   a dental prophylaxis
  b.   curettage
  c.   root planing
  d.   scaling

15. A _____ is used to outline the area for a gingivectomy.
  a.   periodontal knife
  b.   periodontal probe
  c.   pocket marker

16. In charting tooth mobility, Class _____ indicates moderate mobility.
  a.   0
  b.   1
  c.   2
  d.   3

17. During the first 24 hours after a gingivectomy, the patient can expect
_____ .
  a.   bleeding from under the dressing
  b.   mild to moderate pain
  c.   severe pain
  d.   A and C

18. Following scaling and curettage, periodontal dressing _____ placed.
  a.   is
  b.   is not

19. A _____ is performed **only** when periodontal pockets are present.
    a. gingivectomy
    b. gingivoplasty

20. The procedure in which embedded calculus and necrotic cementum is removed from the root surface is known as _____ .
    a. curettage
    b. dental prophylaxis
    c. root planing
    d. scaling

21. The patient with a/an _____ periodontal abscess may complain of throbbing, radiating pain.
    a. acute
    b. chronic

22. Following periodontal surgery, the patient should be instructed to avoid _____ .
    a. alcoholic beverages
    b. citrus fruit
    c. spicy foods
    d. A, B, and C

23. A/An _____ is used primarily to remove large deposits of supra-gingival calculus.
    a. chisel scaler
    b. gracey curette
    c. sickle scaler
    d. universal curette

24. Chlorhexidine oral rinse _____ .
    a. causes temporary brown staining
    b. is an anti-inflammatory agent
    c. is the antibiotic most effective in treating periodontitis
    d. A, B, and C

25. _____ periodontal dressing can be applied directly onto the surgical site without mixing.
    a. Eugenol
    b. Light-cured
    c. Noneugenol

164

Competency 26 - 1 *Assisting During Periodontal Surgery*

Performance Objective: Given an appropriate selection of periodontal surgical instruments, the student will select the instruments and materials required for the surgical procedure specified by the instructor.

Note: *The instructor will specify the type of surgery to be performed and the instruments to be included on the preset tray. The instructor will then role play the dentist performing that surgery. Another student will act as the patient.*

Important: *Study both sides of this sheet before continuing.*

Evaluator #1 (Name/date) _____

Evaluator #2 (Name/date) _____

Evaluator #3 (Name/date) _____

Check box if step was performed correctly.	1st	2nd	3rd
1. Gathered the appropriate supplies as specified for the procedure.	❑	❑	❑
2. Arranged the instruments in the sequence of use.	❑	❑	❑
3. Stated the use of each instrument.	❑	❑	❑
4. Covered the tray to protect it until used.	❑	❑	❑
5. Maintained sterile technique while preparing the tray.	❑	❑	❑
6. Scrubbed hands and put on PPE in preparation for assisting during the procedure.	❑	❑	❑
7. Maintained a clear operating field at all times.	❑	❑	❑
8. Anticipated the dentist's needs throughout the procedure.	❑	❑	❑
9. Maintained patient comfort.	❑	❑	❑
10. Followed the appropriate exposure control measures throughout the procedure.	❑	❑	❑

Notes:

Competency 26 - 1 Instrumentation

Circle the appropriate icons if these items would be used in actual patient care.

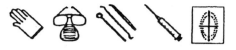

List below all instruments, materials, and supplies required for this procedure.

_____   _____

_____   _____

_____   _____

_____   _____

_____   _____

_____   _____

_____   _____

_____   _____

_____   _____

_____   _____

Competency 26 - 2 *Preparing Periodontal Surgical Dressing*

Performance Objective: The student will demonstrate mixing noneugenol periodontal surgical dressing.

Note: *The instructor will identify the location and extent of the surgical site.*

Important: *Study both sides of this sheet before continuing.*

Evaluator #1 (Name/date) _____

Evaluator #2 (Name/date) _____

Evaluator #3 (Name/date) _____

Check box if step was performed correctly.	1st	2nd	3rd
1. Gathered appropriate supplies.	☐	☐	☐
2. Read and followed the manufacturer's instructions.	☐	☐	☐
3. Dispensed proper amount of material onto mixing pad.	☐	☐	☐
4. Recapped tubes immediately.	☐	☐	☐
5. Thoroughly mixed base and catalyst pastes.	☐	☐	☐
6. Placed mixed material in cup of water.	☐	☐	☐
7. Rolled material into correct length roll.	☐	☐	☐
8. Prepared used supplies for return to the sterilization center.	☐	☐	☐
9. Followed the appropriate exposure control measures throughout the procedure.	☐	☐	☐

Notes:

Competency 26 - 2 Instrumentation
Brand: _____

Circle the appropriate icons if these
items would be used in actual patient
care.

*List below all instruments, materials, and supplies required for this
procedure.*

_____   _____

_____   _____

_____   _____

_____   _____

_____   _____

_____   _____

_____   _____

_____   _____

_____   _____

_____   _____

_____   _____

Chapter 27:
Pediatric Dentistry

Student's Name _____

Learning Objectives

Upon completion of this chapter, the student should be able to:

☐ Describe the services provided in a pediatric dental practice.

☐ Identify the parts of an examination for a child patient and state why each part is important.

☐ List the classifications used to identify the degree of fracture of an anterior tooth.

☐ Describe the process of fabricating a stainless steel crown and state the assistant's role in this procedure.

☐ Discuss the types of pulpal therapy for both primary and young permanent teeth.

☐ If it is legal in your state, demonstrate the topical application of fluoride gel.

☐ If it is legal in your state, demonstrate the application of pit and fissure sealant on an extracted natural tooth.

Exercises

Circle the letter next to the correct answer.

1. The services routinely provided in a pediatric dental office include _____ .
   a. interceptive orthodontics
   b. restorative procedures
   c. surgical procedures
   d. A, B, and C

2. The age groups served by a pediatric dental practice include _____ .
   a. infancy through adolescence
   b. preschool through grade school

3. In a pediatric office, the "quiet room" is used for children _____ .
   a. who are happy patients
   b. who are tired and want to nap
   c. whose behavior may upset other children
   a. A, B, and C

4. Sealants are placed to _____ .
   a. prevent decay on recently erupted teeth
   b. prevent wear on the occlusal surfaces
   c. replace the use of topical fluorides
   d. A, B, and C

5. Trimming and adaptation of a permanent stainless steel crown _____ delegated to the dental assistant.
   a. is
   b. is not

6. The complete removal of the dental pulp that results in a tooth no longer vital is known as a/an _____ .
   a. direct pulp cap
   b. indirect pulp cap
   c. pulpectomy
   d. pulpotomy

7. With a Class _____ fracture of a young anterior tooth, there is an extensive fracture and the pulp is exposed.
   a. 1
   b. 2
   c. 3
   d. 4

8. When selecting a disposable tray for the placement of topical fluoride, a tray that has been tried but did not fit must be _____ .
   a. discarded
   b. disinfected
   c. sterilized

9. The term _____ refers to the treatment of a young permanent tooth that is no longer vital.
   a. apexification
   b. apexogenesis

10. Stainless steel crowns are _____ .
    a. considered to be permanent restorations
    b. indicated when there are rampant caries
    c. used to restore a fractured tooth
    d. A, B, and C

11. The pit and fissure sealant material supplied as a base and a catalyst is _____ .
    a. light-cured
    b. self-cured

170

12. A pit and fissure sealant should **not** be placed if the tooth has _____ .
    a. a well formed occlusal surface
    b. deep pits and fissures
    c. proximal carious lesions
    d. A and C

13. If salivary contamination of the tooth surface occurs after etching, the tooth should be etched again for _____ time period.
    a. half the original
    b. the entire
    c. twice the
    d. None of the above. The tooth should be rinsed, dried and sealed.

14. In an indirect pulp cap procedure, _____ is placed first.
    a. bonding material
    b. calcium hydroxide
    c. zinc oxide and eugenol

15. A crossbite can be corrected with a _____ .
    a. bite plane
    b. fixed space maintainer
    c. mouth guard
    d. removable space maintainer

16. During the examination, very young children may _____ .
    a. allow "fingers only" in their mouth
    b. be seated in the assistant's lap
    c. A and B

17. The teeth most frequently injured by toddlers are the _____ .
    a. mandibular incisors
    b. mandibular molars
    c. maxillary incisors
    d. maxillary molars

18. Traumatic _____ occurs when an injured tooth has been forced inward.
    a. avulsion
    b. extrusion
    c. intrusion
    d. luxation

19. When sizing a stainless steel crown, it must _____ .
    a. allow space for excess cement to escape
    b. fit snugly on the prepared tooth
    c. have both mesial and distal contact
    d. B and C

20. Rubber cup polishing _____ required prior to the application of fluoride gel.
    a. is
    b. is not

21. Rubber cup polishing _____ required prior to etching for the placement of sealants.
    a. is
    b. is not

22. The professional application of fluorides is beneficial for _____ who are at high-risk for caries.
    a. children
    b. adults
    c. A and B

23. Before applying a rinse of topical fluoride, the patient is instructed _____ the solution.
    a. not to swallow
    b. to swallow

24. Mouth guards are fabricated _____ .
    a. of self-cure acrylic
    b. to cover both arches
    c. using the vacuum former
    d. A and B

25. Interceptive orthodontics deals with _____ .
    a. correcting crossbites
    b. correcting oral habits
    c. maintaining space
    d. A, B, and C

172

Competency 27 - 1 *Applying Topical Fluoride Gel*

Performance Objective: The student will demonstrate application of a topical fluoride gel on a patient or typodont.

Note: An assistant is allowed to perform this function **only** in states where it is legal under the rules and regulations of the state dental practice act.

Important: *Study both sides of this sheet before continuing.*

Evaluator #1 (Name/date) _____

Evaluator #2 (Name/date) _____

Evaluator #3 (Name/date) _____

Check box if step was performed correctly.	1st	2nd	3rd
1. Gathered appropriate supplies.	☐	☐	☐
2. Seated patient upright and explained the procedure. Cautioned the patient **not** to swallow the gel.	☐	☐	☐
3. Selected the appropriate tray and lined it with fluoride gel.	☐	☐	☐
4. Dried the teeth using air from the air-water syringe.	☐	☐	☐
5. Inserted the tray and placed the saliva ejector.	☐	☐	☐
6. Set timer for time specified by manufacturer's instructions.	☐	☐	☐
7. Stayed with patient. Upon completion of the treatment removed the tray.	☐	☐	☐
8. Used the HVE tip to remove excess solution from patient's mouth.	☐	☐	☐
9. Maintained patient comfort throughout the treatment.	☐	☐	☐
10. Gave the patient and parent or guardian post treatment instructions.	☐	☐	☐
11. Followed the appropriate exposure control measures throughout the procedure.	☐	☐	☐

Notes:

Competency 27 - 1 Instrumentation

Circle the appropriate icons if these items would be used in actual patient care.

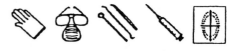

List below all instruments, materials, and supplies required for this procedure.

_____   _____

_____   _____

_____   _____

_____   _____

_____   _____

_____   _____

_____   _____

_____   _____

_____   _____

_____   _____

_____   _____

_____   _____

_____   _____

174

Competency 27 - 2 *Applying Pit and Fissure Sealants*

Performance Objective: The student will demonstrate etching the teeth, applying the sealant, and light curing it. This is to be performed on one or more extracted molars or premolars that have been polished with a fluoride-free abrasive, then rinsed and dried.

Note: An assistant is allowed to perform this function **only** in states where it is specified in the state Dental Practice Act.

Important: *Study both sides of this sheet before continuing.*

Evaluator #1 (Name/date) _____

Evaluator #2 (Name/date) _____

Evaluator #3 (Name/date) _____

Check box if step was performed correctly.	1st	2nd	3rd
1. Gathered appropriate supplies.	☐	☐	☐
2. Stated how teeth have already been polished, rinsed, and thoroughly dried.	☐	☐	☐
3. Described the necessary steps to prevent contamination by moisture or saliva.	☐	☐	☐
4. Placed the etchant on the appropriate surfaces for the time specified by the manufacturer.	☐	☐	☐
5. Rinsed and dried the teeth.	☐	☐	☐
6. Verified the appearance of the etched surface. If not satisfactory, etched surfaces again.	☐	☐	☐
7. Placed the sealant on the etched surfaces.	☐	☐	☐
8. Light cured the material according to the manufacturer's directions.	☐	☐	☐
9. Checked occlusion. Stated how necessary adjustments would be made.	☐	☐	☐
10. Requested that the dentist (instructor) evaluate the completed procedure before the patient was dismissed.	☐	☐	☐
11. Maintained patient comfort through the procedure.	☐	☐	☐
12. Followed the appropriate exposure control measures throughout the procedure.	☐	☐	☐

Notes:

Competency 27 - 2 Instrumentation

Circle the appropriate icons if these items would be used in actual patient care.

List below all instruments, materials, and supplies required for this procedure.

_____   _____

_____   _____

_____   _____

_____   _____

_____   _____

_____   _____

_____   _____

_____   _____

_____   _____

_____   _____

_____   _____

_____   _____

176

Chapter 28:
Orthodontics

Student's Name _____

Learning Objectives

Upon completion of this chapter, the student should be able to:

☐   Describe the factors affecting malocclusion and the phases of orthodontic treatment.

☐   Identify the specialized instruments used in orthodontic treatment.

☐   Identify the diagnostic records that must be gathered before orthodontic treatment planning, including the use of cephalometric radiographs and measurements.

☐   Describe the types of fixed and removable appliances used in orthodontic treatment.

☐   Describe the types and the selection, adaptation, cementation, and removal of orthodontic bands.

☐   Describe the placement and removal of bonded orthodontic brackets.

☐   Demonstrate the placement and removal of elastomeric ring orthodontic separators.

☐   Demonstrate assisting in the cementation of orthodontic bands with zinc phosphate cement.

Exercises

Circle the letter next to the correct answer.

1. When cementing orthodontic bands with zinc phosphate cement, a longer setting time is achieved by _____ .
   a. adding water to the mix
   b. incorporating less powder in the liquid
   c. rapid spatulation of the mix
   d. using an extremely cold, dry slab

2. When serial extractions are required, these are performed by _____ .
   a. an oral surgeon
   b. the referring general dentist
   c. the orthodontist
   d. A or B

3. Indications for orthodontic treatment include _____ .
   a. dysfunction of the temporomandibular joint
   b. impaired mastication
   c. malpositioned teeth
   d. A, B, and C

4. The arch wire is _____ .
   a. a pattern used to align teeth during treatment
   b. attached to labial hooks
   c. bonded directly to the teeth
   d. A and B

5. Elastomeric ties are removed using a/an _____ .
   a. bird beak pliers
   b. explorer
   c. hemostat
   d. orthodontic scaler

6. Dentofacial proportions and the anatomic basis of malocclusion are most effectively evaluated on _____ radiographs.
   a. cephalometric
   b. panoramic

7. The use of orthodontic separators is necessary before placing _____.
   a. arch wires
   b. bands
   c. bonded brackets
   d. ligatures

8. When the maxillary first molars require stabilization or distal movement, _____ is used.
   a. a chin cap
   b. cervical traction
   c. high pull traction

9. To clean under the arch wire, the patient should use _____ .
   a. an interproximal brush
   b. floss
   c. fluoride toothpaste
   d. A and B

10. Once the arch wire is positioned, it is _____ in place.
    a. bonded
    b. ligated

11. There is no vertical overlap of the teeth in an _____ .
    a.   open bite
    b.   overbite
    c.   overjet
    d.   A and B

12. If periodontal problems are present, they are treated _____ orthodontic care is started.
    a.   after
    b.   before

13. On a cephalometric tracing, the _____ is the bottom of the chin.
    a.   basion (Ba)
    b.   gonion (Go)
    c.   menton (Me)
    d.   porion (Po)

14. When there is insurance coverage for orthodontic treatment, it is the responsibility of the _____ to submit periodic progress claims for reimbursement.
    a.   practice
    b.   subscriber

15. The edgewise (buccal) tubes _____ .
    a.   are placed on the lower first molars
    b.   are placed on the upper first molars
    c.   receive the arch wire
    d.   A, B, and C

16. Damage to a tooth bud during development may be a/an _____ cause of malocclusion.
    a.   developmental
    b.   environmental
    c.   genetic

17. To retain the teeth in their position following the removal of the orthodontic bands, the patient wears a/an _____ for 6 to 12 months.
    a.   active retainer
    b.   Hawley retainer
    c.   orthodontic positioner

18. When placing steel separating springs, the spring is slipped into place with the helix to the _____ side of the tooth.
    a.   buccal
    b.   lingual

19. During the final stages of treatment, a/an _____ arch wire is used to position the crown and root in the correct maxillary and mandibular relationship.
    a. flat
    b. nickel titanium
    c. round
    d. square or rectangular

20. Intraoral photographs of orthodontic patients include _____ .
    a. mandibular occlusal view
    b. maxillary occlusal view
    c. right buccal view
    d. A, B, and C

21. Steps taken to correct problems as they are developing are classified as _____ orthodontics.
    a. corrective
    b. interceptive
    c. preventive

22. An orthodontic scaler is used to _____ .
    a. aid in direct bracket placement
    b. remove elastomeric rings
    c. remove excessive cement
    d. A, B, and C

23. In preparation for bonding brackets _____ .
    a. rubber band separators are placed
    b. the teeth are isolated using cotton rolls or retractors
    c. the teeth are polished using a fluoride paste
    d. A, B, and C

24. Before placing an arch wire, the wire is measured _____ .
    a. by the orthodontist
    b. in the patient's mouth
    c. on the patient's diagnostic casts
    d. A and B

25. When preparing to do a cephalometric tracing, the acetate paper is placed rough side _____ over the film.
    a. down
    b. up

180

Competency 28 - 1 *Placing and Removing Orthodontic Separators*

Performance Objective: Using a typodont, the student will demonstrate the placement and removal of elastomeric ring orthodontic separators in preparation for band placement of maxillary first molars.

Important: *Study both sides of this sheet before continuing.*

Evaluator #1 (Name/date) _____

Evaluator #2 (Name/date) _____

Evaluator #3 (Name/date) _____

Check box if step was performed correctly.	1st	2nd	3rd
1. Gathered appropriate supplies.	☐	☐	☐
2. Explained the procedure to the patient.	☐	☐	☐
3. Placed the separator over the beaks of separating pliers.	☐	☐	☐
4. Opened the pliers to stretch the separator ring.	☐	☐	☐
5. Gently forced the ring through the contacts with a seesaw motion.	☐	☐	☐
6. Stated how long this type of separator may be left in place.	☐	☐	☐
7. Selected an orthodontic scaler for removal of the separator.	☐	☐	☐
8. Slipped the scaler tip into the doughnut-shaped separator.	☐	☐	☐
9. Use slight pressure to remove the ring from under the contact.	☐	☐	☐
10. Used an appropriate fulcrum throughout.	☐	☐	☐
11. Maintained patient comfort throughout.	☐	☐	☐
12. Followed the appropriate exposure control measures throughout the procedure.	☐	☐	☐

Notes:

Competency 28 - 1 Instrumentation

Circle the appropriate icons if these items would be used in actual patient care.

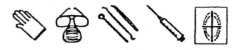

List below all instruments, materials, and supplies required for this procedure.

_____   _____

_____   _____

_____   _____

_____   _____

_____   _____

_____   _____

_____   _____

_____   _____

_____   _____

_____   _____

_____   _____

Competency 28 - 2 *Assisting in the Cementation of Orthodontic Bands*

Performance Objective: The student will demonstrate assisting during this procedure by mixing the cement, loading, and passing the band.

Note: *In states where it is legal, the student may also demonstrate removing excess cement from a typodont.*

Important: *Study both sides of this sheet before continuing.*

Evaluator #1 (Name/date) _____

Evaluator #2 (Name/date) _____

Evaluator #3 (Name/date) _____

Check box if step was performed correctly.	1st	2nd	3rd
1. Gathered appropriate supplies including chilled glass slab.	☐	☐	☐
2. Placed preselected orthodontic band on masking tape.	☐	☐	☐
3. Dispensed cement according to the manufacturer's directions.	☐	☐	☐
4. Replaced covers on containers immediately.	☐	☐	☐
5. Mixed cement according to the manufacturer's directions. to the appropriate consistency.	☐	☐	☐
6. Mix allowed adequate working time.	☐	☐	☐
7. Loaded cement into the band and passed the band to the operator.	☐	☐	☐
8. Passed the band seater to the operator.	☐	☐	☐
9. **Optional:** Demonstrated removal of excess cement while maintaining an appropriate fulcrum throughout.	☐	☐	☐
10. Anticipated the operator's needs throughout.	☐	☐	☐
11. Prepared supplies to be returned to the sterilization area.	☐	☐	☐
12. Followed the appropriate exposure control measures throughout the procedure.	☐	☐	☐

Notes:

Competency 28 - 2 Instrumentation

Brand of Cement _____

Circle the appropriate icons if these
items would be used in actual patient
care.

*List below all instruments, materials, and supplies required for this
procedure.*

_____	_____
_____	_____
_____	_____
_____	_____
_____	_____
_____	_____
_____	_____
_____	_____
_____	_____
_____	_____

Chapter 29:
Endodontics

Student's Name _____

Learning Objectives

Upon completion of this chapter, the student should be able to:

❏   State the indications and contraindications for endodontic treatment.

❏   Identify the specialized instruments used in endodontic treatment.

❏   Describe the specialized diagnostic tests used in an endodontic examination.

❏   Explain why dental dam is required during endodontic treatment.

❏   Discuss the specialized local anesthesia techniques that may be used during endodontic treatment.

❏   Describe the steps in endodontic treatment.

❏   Demonstrate performing a pulp vitality test on a normal tooth using an electric pulp tester.

Exercises

Circle the letter next to the correct answer.

1. The instrument used for the final enlargement of the canal is a _____ .
    a.   barbed broach
    b.   K-type file
    c.   lentulo spiral

2. During endodontic treatment, the canals are irrigated with _____ .
    a.   glutaraldehyde, 2 percent
    b.   iodine mixed with alcohol
    c.   sodium hypochlorite diluted with water
    d.   sterile saline solution

3. Following irrigation, the canals are dried with _____ .
    a.   cotton pellets
    b.   gauze sponges
    c.   paper points
    d.   quick blasts of air

4. During electric pulp testing, the tip is never placed on _____ .
   a. metal restorations
   b. the enamel
   c. the gingiva
   d. A and C

5. After placement and before treatment begins, the dental dam is disinfected with _____ .
   a. alcohol
   b. hydrogen perborate
   c. hydrogen peroxide
   d. sodium hypochlorite

6. A surgical procedure in which the root canal is sealed from the apex is called a/an _____ .
   a. apical curettage
   b. hemisection
   c. inverted
   d. retrograde

7. The prepared canals are filled with _____ .
   a. amalgam
   b. calcium hydroxide
   c. composite
   d. gutta-percha

8. To detect vertical fractures in the crown of the tooth, a _____ may be used.
   a. mobility test
   b. pulp test
   c. thermal test
   d. transillumination

9. In some states, the assistant is allowed to _____ .
   a. expose the trial-point radiograph
   b. place cement into the prepared canal
   c. use a hot instrument to remove excess gutta percha
   d. A, B, and C

10. Endodontic treatment is **not** recommended when the _____ .
    a. diagnosis is reversible pulpitis
    b. patient has a medical condition that precludes any dental treatment
    c. tooth has severe periodontal involvement
    d. A, B, and C

11. During endodontic treatment, local anesthesia may _____ .
    a. be difficult to obtain in the presence of infection
    b. be used selectively as a diagnostic test
    c. not be required when the tooth is nonvital
    d. A, B, and C

12. During pulp testing, if the suspect tooth is the maxillary right first premolar, the control tooth should be the _____ premolar.
    a. mandibular left first
    b. mandibular right first
    c. maxillary left first
    d. maxillary right second

13. A necrotic pulp _____ respond to cold.
    a. will
    b. will not

14. A/An _____ may be required if there is severe periodontal involvement and untreatable bone loss around one of the roots or at the furcation.
    a. apicoectomy
    b. apical curettage
    c. hemisection
    d. none of the above

15. Before treatment, the endodontic patient should be told _____ .
    a. that all root canal treatments are successful
    b. that patients never experience postoperative pain
    c. what the fee will be
    d. A, B, and C

16. An inflammation of the pulp that may be able to heal itself is _____ pulpitis.
    a. irreversible
    b. reversible

17. A _____ is football shaped and is used in a low-speed handpiece.
    a. Gates-Glidden bur
    b. K-type file
    c. lentulo spiral
    d. pesso file

18. A general dentist _____ legally perform endodontic treatment.
    a. may
    b. may not

19. A/An _____ is a double-ended instrument used to remove excess gutta-percha from the crown of the tooth.
    a. endodontic spoon excavator
    b. endodontic spreader
    c. Glick #1
    d. Hedstrom file

20. The standard of care established by the American Dental Association for endodontic treatment requires the use of _____ during endodontic treatment.
    a. antibiotics
    b. dental dam
    c. local anesthesia
    d. A, B, and C

21. An inaccurate canal measurement may result in _____ .
    a. overfilling the canal
    b. perforating the apex
    c. underfilling the canal
    d. A, B, and C

22. Following completed endodontic treatment the _____ places the final restoration.
    a. endodontist
    b. general dentist

23. A/An _____ is the surgical removal of the apical portion of the root.
    a. apical curettage
    b. apicoectomy
    c. hemisection
    d. obturation

24. _____ have tiny fishhook-like barbs along the shaft and are used to remove the bulk of the pulpal tissue.
    a. Broaches
    b. Endodontic explorers
    c. Hedstrom files
    d. None of the above

25. _____ are used in a low-speed handpiece to place sealer and cements into the canals.
    a. Flexible K-type files
    b. Gates-Glidden burs
    c. Lentulo spirals
    d. Pesso files

188

Competency 29 - 1 *Obtaining an Electric Pulp Testing Reading*

Performance Objective: The student will demonstrate obtaining a pulp vitality test reading on a control tooth. A normal (vital) maxillary central incisor is suggested for this purpose.

Important: *Study both sides of this sheet before continuing.*

Evaluator #1 (Name/date) _____

Evaluator #2 (Name/date) _____

Evaluator #3 (Name/date) _____

Check box if step was performed correctly.	1st	2nd	3rd
1. Gathered appropriate supplies.	☐	☐	☐
2. Explained the procedure to the patient.	☐	☐	☐
3. Isolated the tooth to be tested and dried it thoroughly.	☐	☐	☐
4. Placed a small dab of toothpaste on the tip of the pulp tester electrode.	☐	☐	☐
5. Placed the tip of the electrode on the gingival one-third of the facial surface of the tooth to be tested.	☐	☐	☐
6. Started with the setting at zero and gradually increased the setting until the patient responded.	☐	☐	☐
7. Stopped as soon as the patient responded.	☐	☐	☐
8. Recorded the reading on the patient's chart.	☐	☐	☐
9. Maintained patient comfort through the procedure.	☐	☐	☐
10. When finished, prepared supplies for sterilization or return to storage.	☐	☐	☐
11. Followed the appropriate exposure control measures throughout the procedure.	☐	☐	☐

Notes:

Competency 29 - 1 Instrumentation

Circle the appropriate icons if these items would be used in actual patient care.

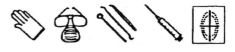

List below all instruments, materials, and supplies required for this procedure.

_____   _____

_____   _____

_____   _____

_____   _____

_____   _____

_____   _____

_____   _____

_____   _____

_____   _____

_____   _____

_____   _____

190

Chapter 30:
Oral and Maxillofacial
Surgery and Dental Implants

Student's Name _____

Learning Objectives

Upon completion of this chapter, the student should be able to:

❏   Explain the difference between a general dentist and an oral and maxillofacial surgeon (OMFS) and list the procedures most commonly performed by an OMFS.

❏   Describe the role of the dental assistant in surgical procedures.

❏   State the difference between incisional and excisional biopsies.

❏   Name the two types of dental implants approved by the American Dental Association (ADA).

❏   Discuss the indications and contraindications for dental implants.

❏   Describe the home care procedures required for dental implants.

❏   Describe the two stages of surgery for placement of osseointegrated dental implants.

❏   Demonstrate identifying the specialized instruments used for common surgical procedures.

Exercises

Circle the letter next to the correct answer.

1.   The indications for dental implants include _____ .
   a.   increasing patient satisfaction for a full lower denture
   b.   providing support for a partial denture
   c.   replacing one or more teeth with single unit crowns
   d.   A, B, and C

2.   In a/an _____ biopsy, the entire lesion is removed.
   a.   excisional
   b.   exfoliative

3. The surgical reshaping of the alveolar ridge is known as a/an _____ .
   a. alveolitis
   b. alveoloplasty
   c. gingivectomy

4. Sutures that are not resorbed by the body are usually removed in _____ days.
   a. 1 to 2
   b. 3 to 4
   c. 5 to 7

5. Dental implants are most frequently made from _____ .
   a. porcelain fused to metal
   b. stainless steel
   c. titanium

6. During oral surgical procedures, _____ may be used for pain control.
   a. conscious sedation
   b. local anesthetic
   c. sedative premedication
   d. A, B, and C

7. Surgical instruments are classified as critical items and must be _____ before reuse.
   a. high-level disinfected
   b. sterilized
   c. A or B is acceptable

8. The function of the rongeur is to _____ .
   a. debride the socket following the extraction
   b. loosen the tooth in the socket
   c. remove the tooth from the socket
   d. trim the alveolar bone

9. Dental implants are contraindicated when _____ is present.
   a. a condition that would interfere with normal healing
   b an irregular bony ridge
   c. dense alveolar bone
   d. A, B, and C

10. Periosteal elevators are used to _____ .
    a. remove clots and debris from the socket following the extraction
    b. remove the tooth from the socket
    c. separate the periosteum from the surface of the bone

11. A/An _____ implant is placed into the bone.
    a. endosteal
    b. subperiosteal
    c. supraosteal

12. Oral surgery is contraindicated when the patient _____ .
    a. has a bleeding or clotting disorder
    b. has poorly controlled diabetes
    c. is taking immunosuppressive drugs
    d. A, B, and C

13. A surgical stent is used to _____ .
    a. help the surgeon place the implants in the proper location
    b. hold the sutures in place
    c. stabilize the bone after surgery

14. When a malignant tumor is diagnosed the patient _____ .
    a. requires immediate treatment by a qualified specialist
    b. should be informed of the biopsy results by the dentist
    c. should be informed of the biopsy results immediately by telephone
    d. A and B

15. All prescriptions given to the patient must be _____ .
    a. approved by the patient's insurance company
    b. approved by the patient's physician
    c. entered in the patient's chart.
    d. B and C

16. The common term for alveolitis is _____ .
    a. dry socket
    b. excessive bleeding
    c. impaction

17. For home care, a dental implant patient may use _____ .
    a. dental implant floss
    b. end-tufted toothbrushes
    c. single-tufted toothbrushes
    d. A, B, and C

18. Many general dentists prefer to _____ .
    a. perform common dental surgical procedures in their practices
    b. refer complex dental surgical procedures to a specialist
    c. A and B

19. In preparation for oral surgery, _____ radiographs are of the **least** value to the surgeon.
    a. bite-wing
    b. extraoral
    c. panoramic
    d. periapical

20. The primary function of a surgical curette is to _____ .
    a. loosen the tooth in the socket
    b. remove the tooth from the socket
    c. scrape the interior of the socket to remove tissue and/or abscesses

21. The bone file is commonly used in surgery after the _____ .
    a. elevator
    b. forceps
    c. hemostat
    d. ronguers

22. A surgical chisel with a bevel on only one side of the edge is used to _____ .
    a. remove tooth
    b. split bone

23. Surgical aspirator tips are _____ those used in restorative dentistry.
    a. much smaller than
    b. slightly larger than
    c. the same size as

24. During a surgical procedure, PPE includes _____ .
    a. examination gloves
    b. overgloves
    c. sterile surgical gloves
    d. B and C

25. Postoperative patient instructions should _____ .
    a. be provided in both written and verbal form
    b. caution the patient about strenuous exercise
    c. explain about biting on a gauze pad
    d. A, B, and C

194

Competency 30 - 1 *Identifying Oral Surgery Instruments*

Performance Objective: Given an assortment of commonly used oral surgery instruments, the student will identify the instruments by type.

Important: *The instructor will select 10 commonly used surgery instruments (of different types) and number them 1 through 10.*

Evaluator #1 (Name/date) _____

Evaluator #2 (Name/date) _____

Evaluator #3 (Name/date) _____

Check box if step was performed correctly.	1st	2nd	3rd
1. Correctly identified instrument #1 as a/an _____.	☐	☐	☐
2. Correctly identified instrument #2 as a/an _____.	☐	☐	☐
3. Correctly identified instrument #3 as a/an _____.	☐	☐	☐
4. Correctly identified instrument #4 as a/an _____.	☐	☐	☐
5. Correctly identified instrument #5 as a/an _____.	☐	☐	☐
6. Correctly identified instrument #6 as a/an _____.	☐	☐	☐
7. Correctly identified instrument #7 as a/an _____.	☐	☐	☐
8. Correctly identified instrument #8 as a/an _____.	☐	☐	☐
9. Correctly identified instrument #9 as a/an _____.	☐	☐	☐
10. Correctly identified instrument #10 as a/an _____.	☐	☐	☐

Notes:

Competency 30 - 2 *Preparing an Instrument Tray for an Extraction*

Performance Objective: Given an appropriate selection of surgical instruments, the student will select the instruments required for a single extraction. The student will state the use of each instrument. Sterile technique must be followed while preparing the tray.

Important: *The instructor will play the role of the dentist and identify the tooth to be extracted and specifying the instruments to be included on the tray. Appropriate PPE must also be available.*

Evaluator #1 (Name/date) _____

Evaluator #2 (Name/date) _____

Evaluator #3 (Name/date) _____

Check box if step was performed correctly.	1st	2nd	3rd
1. Gathered the appropriate supplies as specified on the instructor's instrumentation list.	☐	☐	☐
2. Arranged the instruments in the sequence of use on the tray.	☐	☐	☐
3. Maintained sterile technique while preparing the tray.	☐	☐	☐
4. Stated the use of each instrument.	☐	☐	☐
5. Covered the tray to protect it until used.	☐	☐	☐
6. Followed the appropriate exposure control measures throughout the procedure.	☐	☐	☐

Notes:

Chapter 31:
Fixed Prosthodontics

Student's Name _____

Learning Objectives

Upon completion of this chapter, the student should be able to:

❑   Name indications and contraindications for fixed prosthetics.

❑   Differentiate between noble and base metals and discuss their use in dental alloys.

❑   Describe the differences between full crowns, inlays, onlays, and veneer crowns.

❑   Identify the components of a fixed bridge.

❑   Describe the function of temporary coverage for a fixed bridge.

❑   Describe the use of retraction cord prior to taking a final impression.

❑   Discuss the uses of core build-ups, pins, and posts in crown retention.

❑   Demonstrate creating provisional coverage for a tooth with a crown preparation.

Exercises

Circle the letter next to the correct answer.

1.   In a fixed bridge, the replacement for a natural tooth is called a/an _____ .
   a.   abutment
   b.   clasp
   c.   pontic
   d.   retainer

2.   A cast restoration that covers most of the occlusal surface and the proximal surfaces is known as an _____ .
   a.   inlay
   b.   onlay

3. The noble metals used in dentistry are _____ .
   a. gold, platinum, and silver
   b. gold, palladium, and platinum
   c. gold, platinum, and silver
   d. gold and silver

4. The measure of stress before fracture occurs in a material is called _____ strength.
   a. elongation
   b. hardness
   c. tensile
   d. yield

5. When fitting a temporary aluminum crown, the first measurement is of the _____ space.
   a. mesial-to-distal
   b. lingual-to-acial

6. When selecting the shade for a porcelain veneer, the color of the finished veneer is influenced by the shade of the _____ .
   a. luting agent
   b. underlying tooth structure
   c. A and B

7. When creating custom temporary coverage, an alginate impression is taken _____ the tooth is prepared.
   a. after
   b. before

8. Gingival retraction cord containing epinephrine _____ .
   a. causes the desired temporary tissue shrinkage
   b. is contraindicated for patients with cardiovascular disease
   c. is used to control bleeding
   d. A, B, and C

9. To strengthen the retention of a cast crown on a vital tooth, a _____ may be placed.
   a. core build-up and retention pins
   b. post, core build-up, and retention pins
   c. post and retention pins

10. When a restoration is constructed in the dental laboratory, the _____ technique is used.
    a. direct
    b. indirect

11. When fitting a preformed acrylic crown, the height is reduced by using _____ the cervical margin.
    a. an acrylic bur to smooth
    b. contouring pliers to shape
    c. crown scissors to trim

12. In a bridge, the replacement teeth are supported by _____ .
    a. abutments
    b. clasps
    c. retainers
    d. A or C

13. In a _____ crown, the natural enamel on the facial surface is visible and the prepared portion is covered by the crown.
    a. acrylic
    b. porcelain-fused-to-metal
    c. three-quarter
    d. veneer

14. When placing retraction cord, the operator usually tucks the cord into the sulcus, working in a _____ direction.
    a. clockwise
    b. counterclockwise

15. Temporary coverage is acceptable when the _____ .
    a. cervical margin is smooth and fits snugly
    b. contours are similar to those of the natural tooth
    c. occlusal surface is aligned with the occlusal plane of the adjacent teeth
    d. A, B, and C

16. Temporary coverage may be cemented in place with _____ .
    a. glass ionomer cement
    b. IRM with a small amount of petroleum jelly added
    c. zinc phosphate cement
    d. A or B

17. After the teeth have been prepared for porcelain veneers, temporary coverage _____ .
    a. is required because the teeth are very sensitive
    b. is not required because only a thin layer of enamel has been removed

18. A _____ bridge requires very little preparation of the abutment teeth and the completed restoration is bonded in place.
     a. fixed
     b. Maryland
     c. resin bonded bridge
     d. B and C

19. As part of his home care plan the patient with a fixed bridge is _____ .
     a. instructed never to disturb the area under the pontic
     b. taught how to floss under the pontic

20. A wooden bite stick is used to _____ .
     a. aid in removing the temporary coverage
     b. completely seat a cast restoration
     c. register the occlusion of the cast restoration

21. Before sending the case to the dental laboratory for construction of a bridge, the _____ .
     a. bite registration must be obtained
     b. dentist must write the laboratory prescription
     c. final impression and opposing arch impression must be obtained
     d. A, B, and C

22. A high noble alloy must contain at least _____ percent noble metals.
     a. 40
     b. 50
     c. 60
     d. 100

23. When the dentist is preparing a tooth for a full crown, the _____ of the tooth is/are reduced.
     a. contour
     b. height
     c. A and B

24. During the try-in visit for a bridge, if the castings fit _____ .
     a. an impression is taken with the castings in place
     b. the castings are removed and a final impression is taken
     c. the castings are temporarily cemented in place

25. Custom temporary coverage is constructed of _____ .
     a. light-cured composite
     b. self-cured acrylic
     c. self-curied composite

200

Competency 31 - 1 *Creating Provisional Coverage*

Performance Objective: In states where it is legal, the student will create a temporary acrylic crown for a molar with a full crown preparation. This will be performed on a typodont or mannikin.

Important: *Study both sides of this sheet before continuing.*

Evaluator #1 (Name/date) _____

Evaluator #2 (Name/date) _____

Evaluator #3 (Name/date) _____

Check box if step was performed correctly.	1st	2nd	3rd
1. Gathered appropriate supplies.	☐	☐	☐
2. Obtained an acceptable alginate impression before the tooth was prepared.	☐	☐	☐
3. Mixed the acrylic monomer and polymer.	☐	☐	☐
4. Coated the prepared tooth with petroleum jelly or separating medium.	☐	☐	☐
5. Placed the prepared acrylic dough into the impression in the area of the prepared tooth.	☐	☐	☐
6. Placed the impression back in the "patient's" mouth.	☐	☐	☐
7. Allowed the material to reach initial set.	☐	☐	☐
8. Removed the tray from the patient's mouth and removed the temporary covering from the impression.	☐	☐	☐
9. Trimmed excess material from the margins of the temporary covering.	☐	☐	☐
10. Replaced the temporary covering on the prepared tooth and left it there until setting was complete.	☐	☐	☐
11. Removed and evaluated the temporary coverage including the margins.	☐	☐	☐
12. If the margins and/or the temporary were not acceptable, started over.	☐	☐	☐
13. Smoothed the edges, made necessary adjustments, and completed the crown.	☐	☐	☐
14. Followed the appropriate exposure control measures throughout the procedure.	☐	☐	☐

Notes:

Competency 31 - 1 Instrumentation

Circle the appropriate icons if these items would be used in actual patient care.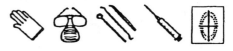

List below all instruments, materials, and supplies required for this procedure.

_____ _____

_____ _____

_____ _____

_____ _____

_____ _____

_____ _____

_____ _____

_____ _____

_____ _____

_____ _____

_____ _____

Student's Name _____

Learning Objectives

Upon completion of this chapter, the student should be able to:

☐ Differentiate between a complete and partial denture.

☐ Describe the indications and contraindications for removable partial and complete dentures.

☐ List the components of a partial and complete denture.

☐ Describe the steps in the construction of a removable partial denture.

☐ Discuss the steps in the construction of a complete denture.

☐ Describe the construction of an overdenture and an immediate denture.

☐ Describe the process of relining or repairing a complete or partial denture.

☐ Demonstrate taking an alginate impression on edentulous mandibular and maxillary arches.

Exercises

Circle the letter next to the correct answer.

1. The choice of a removable prosthesis is influenced by the patient's _____ .
   a. attitude toward replacing lost teeth
   b. mental health
   c. physical health
   d. A, B, and C

2. To provide good support for a removable prosthesis, the alveolar ridge should be _____ .
   a. thick
   b. high
   c. thin
   d. B and C

3. A prosthesis is always _____ before it is placed in the patient's mouth.
   a. disinfected
   b. sterilized

4. The framework for a removable partial denture is usually constructed of a _____ alloy.
   a. base metal
   b. gold
   c. high noble
   d. noble metal

5. The saddle of a removable partial denture _____ .
   a. holds the artificial teeth
   b. provides some support for the prosthesis
   c. rests on the oral mucosa covering the alveolar ridge
   d. A, B, and C

6. During the baseplate-occlusal rim try-in, the dentist records the _____ .
   a. cuspid eminence
   b. occlusal relationships
   c. smile line
   d. A, B, and C

7. Retention for a maxillary full denture depends primarily on suction seal created by the _____ .
   a. alveolar ridge
   b. post dam

8. The right and left quadrant framework of the partial denture are joined by a _____ .
   a. clasp
   b. connector
   c. retainer
   d. saddle

9. Artificial teeth for a complete denture usually _____ include third molars.
   a. do
   b. do not

10. Because of their relatively weak root structure, individual _____ are the least acceptable teeth for use as abutments.
    a. cuspids
    b. incisors
    c. premolars
    d. third molars

11. Acrylic artificial teeth may be selected because they _____ .
    a. do not produce a clicking sound during mastication
    b. wear well under stress
    c. A and B

12. Posterior denture teeth are retained by _____ .
    a. cementing them to the base
    b. gold pins in the back of the tooth
    c. saddle acrylic flowed into a hole in the base of the tooth
    d. welding the tooth to the frame

13. The alginate-hydrocolloid impression technique uses _____ .
    a. a custom tray
    b. fast-setting alginate
    c. syringe-type hydrocolloid impression material
    c. A, B, and C

14. A surgical template for an immediate denture is used to _____ .
    a. detect pressure points on the alveolar ridge
    b. take the final impression
    c. verify the shape of the alveolar ridge
    d. A and C

15. When preparing teeth for an overdenture, a short coping technique is used with _____ teeth.
    a. badly worn
    b. endodontically treated
    c. vital
    d. A and C

16. The mandible placed as far forward as possible from the centric position is known as _____ .
    a. lateral excursion
    b. protrusion
    c. retrusion

17. When a denture is to be relined in the laboratory, the impression is taken using _____ .
    a. a custom tray
    b. a perforated stock tray
    c. a solid stock tray
    d. the patient's current denture

18. When selecting artificial teeth, the _____ number designates the shape of the teeth.
    a. mold
    b. size

19. In a partial denture, a precision attachment _____ of the saddle.
    a. prevents lateral movement
    b. provides stabilization
    c. provides vertical movement
    d. A and C

20. The extent of seating of a prosthesis is controlled by a _____ .
    a. clasp
    b. connector
    c. rest
    d. retainer

21. Taking an alginate impression of an edentulous arch differs from taking impressions of arches with teeth because _____ .
    a. an edentulous tray is used
    b. more extensive tissue details are needed
    c. the height of the teeth is missing
    d. A, B, and C

22. During the _____ try-in the patient is asked to make *f, v, s,* and *th* sounds.
    a. baseplate-occlusal rim
    b. wax set-up

23. The occlusal relationship for a complete denture is recorded _____ .
    a. using elastomeric impression material
    b. using the functionally generated path technique
    c. when the final impression is taken
    d. A and C

24. A prosthesis to be returned to the laboratory is disinfected by _____ .
    a. soaking it in dilute isopropyl alcohol
    b. soaking it in an EPA-registered disinfectant
    c. spraying it with an EPA-registered disinfectant
    d. B and/or C

25. For the delivery of a partial denture, an appointment of _____ minutes is usually adequate.
    a. 10 to 20
    b. 20 to 30
    c. 30 to 45
    d. 45 to 60

Competency 32 - 1 *Taking Alginate Impressions of Edentulous Arches*

Performance Objective: Working with edentulous models or stone diagnostic casts, the student will demonstrate taking an alginate impression of an edentulous mandibular arch and an edentulous maxillary arch.

Note: This procedure is to be performed only in those states where it is legal.

Important: *Study both sides of this sheet before continuing.*

Evaluator #1 (Name/date) _____

Evaluator #2 (Name/date) _____

Evaluator #3 (Name/date) _____

Check box if step was performed correctly.	1st	2nd	3rd
1. Gathered appropriate supplies.	☐	☐	☐
2. Explained the procedure to the patient.	☐	☐	☐
Mandibular arch:			
3. Selected an appropriate tray.	☐	☐	☐
4. Modified edges of tray with wax.	☐	☐	☐
5. Mixed material and seated impression.	☐	☐	☐
6. Described the use of fingers to gently massage the area of the face over the borders of the tray.	☐	☐	☐
7. Removed and evaluated the completed impression.	☐	☐	☐
Maxillary arch:			
8. Selected an appropriate tray.	☐	☐	☐
9. Modified edges of tray with wax.	☐	☐	☐
10. Mixed material and seated impression.	☐	☐	☐
11. Described the use of fingers to gently massage the area of the face over the borders of the tray.	☐	☐	☐
12. Removed and evaluated the completed impression.	☐	☐	☐
13. Followed the appropriate exposure control measures throughout the procedure.	☐	☐	☐

Notes:

Competency 32 - 1 Instrumentation

Circle the appropriate icons if these items would be used in actual patient care.

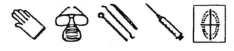

List below all instruments, materials, and supplies required for this procedure.

_____   _____

_____   _____

_____   _____

_____   _____

_____   _____

_____   _____

_____   _____

_____   _____

_____   _____

_____   _____

208

Chapter 33:
Business Office Management

Student's Name _____

Learning Objectives

Upon completion of this chapter, the student should be able to:

☐ Describe how marketing applies to a dental practice and differentiate between internal and external marketing.

☐ Discuss the steps in outlining the appointment book and in making appointment entries.

☐ Describe how to schedule appointments for the following: children, emergency patients, new patients, recall patients, and utilizing an EFDA.

☐ Identify how to use these filing systems: alphabetical, numerical, cross-reference, chronological, and subject.

☐ Name three types of preventive recall systems and state the benefits of each.

☐ Demonstrate professional telephone courtesy.

☐ Demonstrate the proper procedure for greeting patients.

Exercises

Circle the letter next to the correct answer.

1. Treatment for Mrs. Harris was completed in September. With a 6 month recall period, she should be reappointed again in _____ .
   a. April
   b. August
   c. March
   d. November

2. The appointment book entry is made _____ the appointment card is completed.
   a. after
   b. before

3. A system that enables one to locate materials filed under numerical filing is known as a/an _____ file.
   a. alphabetical
   b. chronological
   c. cross-reference
   d. tickler

4. The patient's clinical records are _____ .
   a. always retained in the active file
   b. considered to be permanent records
   c. never discarded without the dentist's permission
   d. B and C

5. Most practices work on a _____ minute time unit system because it provides scheduling flexibility.
   a. 5
   b. 10
   c. 15
   d. 30

6. To make it easier to sort records into active and inactive files _____ are used.
   a. file dividers
   b. outguides
   c. purge tabs

7. New patients are _____ .
   a. asked to come 15 minutes before their appointment
   b. placed on a waiting list
   c. scheduled as soon as possible
   d. A and C

8. Computerized files are protected by making a _____ copy.
   a. back-up
   b. print

9. Outlining the appointment book involves entering information concerning _____ .
   a. buffer periods
   b. holidays
   c. times when the office is closed
   d. A, B, and C

10. The dentist will usually speak on the telephone to _____ .
    a. new patients
    b. his or her immediate family members
    c. out-of-state sales representatives
    d. A and B

11. When filing alphabetically, titles such as Mrs. and Ph.D. _____ indexing units.
    a. are
    b. are not

12. When scheduling with an EFDA, a dark bar on the left side of the appointment column indicates time when the _____ is with the patient.
    a. dental assistant
    b. dentist
    c. EFDA
    d. registered dental hygienist

13. On the daily schedule form a checkmark next to the patient's name indicates that the _____ .
    a. appointment has been confirmed
    b. appointment has not been confirmed
    c. patient has agreed to pay cash
    d. A and C

14. Publishing a practice newsletter is a form of _____ marketing.
    a. external
    b. internal

15. A broken appointment is recorded on the _____ .
    a. account ledger card
    b. patient's treatment record
    c. A and B

16. The amount of time reserved for a dental hygiene patient is _____ .
    a. 30 minutes
    b. based on the procedure to be performed
    c. based on whether the patient is an adult or a child
    d. B and C

17. A patient with an acute emergency is seen _____ .
    a. at the first cancellation
    b. during buffer time
    c. immediately

18. All appointment book entries are made in _____ .
    a. ink
    b. pencil

19. When making a recording on an office telephone answering machine, the business manger should _____ .
    a. give dentist's home telephone number
    b. speak slowly and clearly
    c. state how to reach the doctor in the event of a dental emergency
    d. B and C

20. Accounts receivable records, expenses, business correspondence, and payroll records are all examples of _____ records.
    a. non-clinical
    b. patient financial
    c. practice
    d. tax

21. With effective appointment control _____ .
    a. patients are seen on time
    b. the dentist and staff make effective use of their time
    c. the patient load is well-balanced
    d. A, B, and C

22. It is courteous to permit the person _____ the call to hang up first.
    a. originating
    b. receiving

23. An arriving patient should be _____ .
    a. addressed by his or her first name
    b. greeted promptly and pleasantly
    c. informed of the approximate waiting time
    d. B and C

24. The type of patient record filing system most commonly used in a large practice is a _____ system.
    a. alphabetical
    b. numerical

25. Arrange the following names in correct alphabetical order.

    (1) Wanda Black   (3) George D. Blaine Jr.

    (2) William B. Blake Sr.   (4) G. D. Blaine
    a. 1, 2, 3, 4
    b. 2, 3, 4, 1
    c. 1, 4, 3, 2
    d. 4, 3, 1, 2

Competency 33 - 1 *Making Telephone Calls in a Professional Manner*

Performance Objective: In a classroom simulation, the student will demonstrate calling a patient to confirm his dental appointment. Another student will play the patient.

Note: *The class discussion replaces the use of individual evaluators.*

The assistant knows:
The patient is Ms. Chapman, a very busy businesswoman.
The assistant is calling to confirm Ms. Chapman's appointment.
This is scheduled at 9 AM tomorrow for a crown preparation.

The patient knows:
She is very busy now and would prefer not to be interrupted.
She is working on an important report that must be completed by noon tomorrow.
She is not at all sure that she can keep the appointment tomorrow morning.

Check box if the step was performed correctly.

1. Greeted the patient pleasantly.
   Determined that he or she had reached Ms. Chapman. ☐

2. The assistant identified himself or herself appropriately. ☐

3. The assistant briefly stated the reason for the call. ☐

4. Took the appropriate steps when Ms. Chapman stated
   that she might not be able to keep the appointment. ☐

5. If appropriate, scheduled a new appointment for
   Ms. Chapman. ☐

6. Closed the conversation pleasantly and promptly. ☐

7. Allowed Ms. Chapman to hang up first. ☐

8. Managed the conversation in a professional manner. ☐

9. Achieved the goal of either confirming
   or rescheduling the appointment. ☐

Notes:

Competency 33 - 2 *Greeting an Arriving Patient*

Performance Objective: In a classroom simulation, the student will greet an arriving new patient, Maria Garcia, and ask her to complete a new patient registration and medical history form. Mrs. Garcia has brought her two small children with her. Other students play the roles of Mrs. Garcia and the children.

Note: The class discussion replaces the use of individual evaluators.

The assistant knows:
Mrs. Garcia seems upset.
She seems to speak English well, yet does not want to complete the registration and medical history forms.

The patient knows:
She is very nervous about coming to a new dentist.
She is upset because her baby-sitter did not show up this morning.
She is bilingual, but does not want to fill out "confusing paperwork" because she does not understand the questions.

Check box if step was performed correctly

1. Greeted the patient pleasantly and
    verified the patient's identity.   ❒

2. The assistant introduced him- or herself and
    welcomed Mrs. Garcia to the practice.   ❒

3. Explained the need for the information.
    Asked Mrs. Garcia to complete the required forms.   ❒

4. Suggested that there were toys available to amuse the
    children while Mrs. Garcia did this.   ❒

5. When Mrs. Garcia expressed difficulty completing
    the forms, offered to aid her in completing them.   ❒

6. Maintained a pleasant and professional attitude
    throughout the discussion.   ❒

At this point, stop the role play and discuss how the problem of caring for the children should be handled while Mrs. Garcia is being seen by the dentist.

Notes:

Chapter 34:
Accounts Receivable Management

Student's Name _____

Learning Objectives

Upon completion of this chapter, the student should be able to:

❏   Describe the basic components of both manual and computerized accounts receivable management systems.

❏   Discuss the role of the office manager/business assistant in making financial arrangements and in preventive account management.

❏   List at least three different types of dental insurance plans and describe the factors that limit the patient's benefits under these plans.

❏   Discuss the steps in claims preparation, the use of American Dental Association procedure codes, and the application of the birthday rule when children have dual coverage.

❏   Demonstrate making financial arrangements with a patient

❏   Demonstrate making a telephone collection call on an overdue account.

Exercises

Circle the letter next to the correct answer.

1. Money from the change fund is _____ .
    a.   a variable amount depending upon the day's transactions
    b.   included in the daily deposit
    c.   removed from the drawer at the end of the day
    d.   A and C

2. When a child has dual dental insurance coverage, under the birthday rule, the carrier of the parent _____ is primary.
    a.   who is older
    b.   whose birthday is earlier in the year

3. Electronic claims _____ .
    a.   are submitted via modem
    b.   reduce the possibility of clerical errors
    c.   use information that is already in the practice computer
    d.   A, B, and C

4. You are establishing a divided payment plan for Ms. Browne. The total fee for her treatment will be $1,300. She made a down payment of $400 today. The balance is to be paid in 3 equal payments of $ _____ each.
   a. 300
   b. 400
   c. 433
   d. 567

5. Cosmetic dentistry is an example of treatment that is commonly _____ under a dental insurance plan.
   a. an exclusion
   b. available after the deductible has been met
   c. must not exceed the annual maximum
   d. requires a pre-treatment estimate

6. When tracking and taking action on overdue accounts, a/an _____ report is helpful.
   a. accounts receivable
   b. daily journal
   c. monthly production summary

7. A patient who did not make a payment today may be given a/an _____ .
   a. receipt
   b. walk-out statement

8. _____ are used to transmit fee information from the treatment room to the business office.
   a. Charge slips
   b. Encounter forms
   c. A or B

9. When using a manual bookkeeping system, the account record (showing the amounts charged, paid, and owed) is maintained on the _____ .
   a. account ledger card
   b. patient's chart
   c. A and B

10. A method of tracking the accuracy and completeness of bookkeeping records is known as a/an _____ .
    a. audit trail
    b. restrictive endorsement

11. Eighty percent coinsurance means that the carrier will pay _____ percent of the covered fee and the patient pays the balance.
    a. 20
    b. 80

216

12. Financial arrangements should be made with the patient _____.
    a. at the conclusion of treatment
    b. before the first statement
    c. before treatment begins
    d. when the patient asks

13. The person who represents the family unit in relation to the dental plan is known as the _____.
    a. insured
    b. spouse
    c. subscriber
    d. A or C

14. When a person starts a new job that includes dental insurance, benefits usually begin _____.
    a. after a 30 to 60 day waiting period
    b. after 2 years of employment
    c. immediately
    d. with the first paycheck

15. When a patient makes a payment by credit card, the amount of the bank service charge _____ the balance of the patient's account.
    a. does not change
    b. is added to
    c. is subtracted from

16. The patient signs a/an _____ form, giving the dentist permission to send information concerning his treatment to the insurance company.
    a. attending dentist's statement
    b. assignment of benefits
    c. authorization
    d. release of information

17. Under a/an _____ payment plan, the amount paid by the carrier is based, in part, on the dentist's fee schedule.
    a. HMO
    b. schedule of benefits
    c. UCR

18. Under a/an _____ plan, the employer reimburses the employee for dental expenses.
    a. individual capitation
    b. direct reimbursement
    c. HMO
    d. IPA

19. The insurance codes found in the *Current Dental Terminology* are _____ .
    a. updated periodically
    b. used to report dental treatment to the insurance carrier
    c. very specific and not interchangeable
    d. A, B, and C

20. Mr. Jackson has a policy with a least expensive alternative treatment clause. He requires a fixed bridge, which will cost $3,000. A partial denture to replace these teeth would cost $750. Mr. Jackson's carrier will _____ .
    a. base payment on the fee for the fixed bridge
    b. base payment on the fee for the partial denture
    c. not permit the bridge to be placed
    d. B and C

21. With dual coverage under a _____ plan, the patient will receive total payment not to exceed 100% of the actual fee.
    a. coordination of benefits
    b. nonduplication of benefits

22. Overdue accounts may be collected by _____ .
    a. a collection agency
    b. a collection call
    c. small claims settlement in favor of the dentist
    d. A, B, or C

23. A list of specific amounts the carrier will pay toward the cost of dental services rendered is known as a _____ .
    a. schedule of allowances
    b. schedule of benefits
    c. table of allowances
    d. A, B, and C

24. A/An _____ is an administrative procedure whereby the dentist submits the treatment plan to the carrier before treatment is started.
    a. alternative treatment provision
    b. determination of eligibility
    c. electronic claim
    d. pre-treatment estimate

25. If the patient is not available to sign the insurance claim form, the office manager may _____ .
    a. send the claim to the patient for his signature
    b. sign the form for the patient
    c. type in signature on file
    d. type in signature on request

218

Competency 34 - 1 *Making Financial Arrangements*

Performance Objective: In a classroom simulation, the student will demonstrate making financial arrangements with a new patient. The patient is Mrs. DiNatale. Another student will role play Mrs. DiNatale.

Note: The class discussion replaces the use of individual evaluators.

The assistant knows:
The estimate for Mrs. DiNatale family's dental care is $2,000.
Dr. Schein offers several payment plans. These include accepting credit cards, arranging a bank loan, or arranging a divided payment plan that does not extend beyond 6 months.

The patient knows:
A dental bill of this size is difficult for her because she has 4 children.
She wants to extend her payments out as long as possible.

Check box if step was performed correctly

1. Explained the need for treatment to Mrs. DiNatale. ☐

2. Explained the available payment plans to Mrs. DiNatale. ☐

3. Answered Mrs. DiNatale's questions politely and completely. ☐

4. Arrived at an acceptable agreement with Mrs. DiNatale. ☐

5. Asked Mrs. DiNatale to complete the necessary forms. ☐

6. Maintained a pleasant and professional attitude throughout the discussion. ☐

Notes:

Competency 34 - 2 *Making a Collection Telephone Call*

Performance Objective: In a classroom simulation, the student will demonstrate making a telephone collection call. The call is to Mrs. Moses, who has fallen behind on her payments. Another student will play Mrs. Moses.

Note: The class discussion replaces the use of individual evaluators.

The assistant knows:
Dr. Brown is concerned but willing to work with Mrs. Moses to help her meet this financial commitment.
The amount owed is $500 and no payment has been made in 2 months.

The patient knows:
She is late with the payments because her husband lost his job 3 months ago. He is starting a new job next week.

Check box if step was performed correctly

1. Stated at what hour the phone call was being placed. ☐

2. Determined that she was speaking to the responsible party (Mrs. Moses). ☐

3. Identified herself, her employer, and the reason for the call. ☐

4. Was polite, empathetic, and offered to help. ☐

5. Worked out alternative payment arrangement with Mrs. Moses. ☐

6. Maintained a professional attitude throughout the conversation. ☐

7. Terminated the conversation pleasantly. ☐

8. Recorded the arrangements for the alternative payment plan on the patient's financial record. ☐

Notes:

Chapter 35:
Accounts Payable Management

Student's Name _____

Learning Objectives

Upon completion of this chapter, the student should be able to:

☐ Describe the accounts payable management functions in the dental office, including the procedures for handling COD deliveries and petty cash.

☐ Discuss how to manage inventory control, how to establish the reorder point, and reorder quantity for a specified dental supply item.

☐ State the four factors that should be checked prior to making an equipment service repair call.

☐ State the proper way to handle an NSF check and describe the steps required to make the necessary adjustments in the practice and patient account records.

☐ Identify common payroll taxes, describing which are withheld from the employee's pay, which are the financial responsibility of the employer, and which require matching contributions.

☐ Describe the steps in reconciling a bank statement.

Exercises

Circle the letter next to the correct answer.

1. All practice income, minus payment of all practice-related expenses, yields the dentist's _____ income.
   a. fixed
   b. gross
   c. net
   d. variable

2. A _____ notice is sent to the dentist as notification that an item is not available for delivery with the balance of the order.
   a. back order
   b. bar code
   c. debit memo
   d. purchase order

3. Small practice expenses are paid from the _____ fund.
   a. change
   b. petty cash

4. If it is lost or stolen, a check with a _____ endorsement cannot be cashed.
   a. blanket
   b. dated
   c. personal
   d. restrictive

5. The reorder point for any supply is based on the _____ and the necessary lead time.
   a. back order
   b. inventory system
   c. rate of use
   d. reorder quantity

6. In a large group practice, a/an _____ is a formal application for supplies.
   a. acquisition
   b. inventory request
   c. purchase order
   d. requisition

7. A supply, such as impression material, which is literally "used up" as part of its function, is known as a/an _____ .
   a. consumable
   b. expendable
   c. nonexpendable
   d. A and C

8. Those expenses that continue at all times are known as _____ .
   a. accounts payable
   b. accounts receivable
   c. fixed overhead
   d. variable overhead

9. When balancing a checkbook, those deposits that have been made but are not yet credited to the bank account are known as _____ .
   a. credit memos
   b. debit memos
   c. deposits in transit

10. _____ is **not** a federal payroll deduction.
    a. FICA
    b. FUTA
    c. Income tax
    d. Workers Compensation

11. Before making a service repair call the assistant should check the _____ .
    a. electrical plug
    b. fuse
    c. reset button
    d. A, B, and C

12. Examples of payroll deductions that require a matching contribution by the employer include _____ .
    a. FICA
    b. FUTA
    c. income tax
    d. A and B

13. Within 30 days of the end of the calendar year, or upon termination of employment, the employee must be furnished with a/an _____ form.
    a. Circular E
    b. income tax
    c. W-2
    d. W-4

14. If a NSF check cannot be redeposited, the amount of the check must be _____ the practice's bank balance and income figures.
    a. added to
    b. subtracted from

15. At least once every _____ , the assistant should request a "Statement of Earnings" from the Social Security Administration.
    a. 6 months
    b. 2 years
    c. 3 years
    d. 5 years

16. Promptly after receipt of the bank statement, it should be reconciled with the _____ .
    a. accounts payable records
    b. check register
    c. expense records
    d. A and C

17. The person named on the check as the intended recipient of the amount shown is the _____ .
    a. bearer
    b. maker
    c. payee
    d. payer

18. The amount shown on a paycheck reflects the employee's _____ pay.
    a. gross
    b. net

19. A/An _____ is a form authorizing the purchase of specific supplies from a specific supplier.
    a. invoice
    b. packing slip
    c. purchase order
    d. requisition

20. _____ is a payroll deduction based on earnings and the number of exemptions claimed by the employee.
    a. Federal income tax
    b. FICA
    c. FUTA
    d. Workers compensation

21. When an NSF check cannot be redeposited, the amount of the check is _____ the patient's account balance.
    a. added to
    b. subtracted from

22. _____ are items, other than canceled checks, that have been deducted directly from the checking account.
    a. Credits
    b. Debits

23. The _____ is the maximum amount of a product to be ordered at one time.
    a. inventory quantity
    b. purchase point
    c. reorder point
    d. reorder quantity

24. When using the order tag system _____ should be included on the file card for each product.
    a. applicable descriptive information
    b. full brand name
    c. reorder point and purchase source
    d. A, B, and C

25. _____ ensure the practice a constant supply of an item without bulk storage problems.
    a. Automatic shipments
    b. Bulk ordering
    c. Purchase requisitions
    d. A, B, and C

Chapter 36:
Employment

Student's Name _____

Learning Objectives

Upon completion of this chapter, the student should be able to:

☐   Identify at least three sources where a dental assistant may find information about potential employment opportunities.

☐   Describe at least three types of employment opportunities for the dental assistant

☐   Describe suitable attire for an employment interview.

☐   Identify two important functions when greeting or being dismissed by the interviewer.

☐   Describe the responsibilities of the employee and the employer in maintaining employment in the dental office.

☐   Discuss the elements of an employment agreement.

☐   Demonstrate being interviewed for a position as a chairside assistant.

Exercises

Circle the letter next to the correct answer.

1. The majority of dental offices in the United States are _____ .
   a. group practices
   b. public health clinics
   c. solo private practices
   d. specialty practices

2. References _____ be included in a résumé.
   a. should
   b. should not

3. The benefits to the dental assistant of being employed in a large group practice include _____.
   a. greater opportunity for advancement
   b. opportunities to develop more specialized skills
   c. professional stimulation with other auxiliaries
   d. A, B, and C

4. A legal arrangement between two or more persons having equal rights and duties is called a/an _____ .
   a. expense-sharing arrangement
   b. partnership
   c. professional association
   d. professional corporation

5. All employees of a professional corporation, including the dentists, are subject to _____ .
   a. ADA guidelines
   b. CDC regulations
   c. OSHA regulations
   d. A and C

6. Public health and other government-supported dental clinics may function at the _____ level.
   a. county
   b. federal
   c. state
   d. A, B, and C

7. Civilian dental assistants may be hired under Civil Service to work in _____ .
   a. military installations
   b. Veterans' Administration hospitals
   c. A and/or B

8. As the minimal educational level for a dental assisting instructor, most schools require a _____ .
   a. bachelor's degree
   b. certified or registered dental assistant
   c. master's degree
   d. A and B

9. When responding by telephone to a newspaper classified advertisement about a job, the dental assistant might expect to speak to the _____ .
   a. administrative assistant/office manager
   b. dental hygienist
   e. dentist

10. A statement of your employment objective should be included in your _____ .
    a. letter of application
    b. résumé

11. When employment is secured using their services, a fee is charged by
    _____ .
    a. campus placement bureaus
    b. federal and state government employment bureaus
    c. private employment agencies
    d. A and C

12. Professional information about the applicant is included in the _____ .
    a. interview follow-up letter
    b. letter of application
    c. résumé

13. The business or yellow pages of the telephone directory supply information
    about _____ in the area.
    a. dentists in general and specialty practice
    b. the income potential of a dental assistant
    c. the scope of employment potential
    d. A and C

14. If you are over 19 the interviewer _____ legally ask your age.
    a. may
    b. may not

15. Most employers routinely consider the first several weeks of employment as a
    _____ period.
    a. dormant
    b. permanent
    c. provisional
    d. temporary

16. The *Americans with Disabilities Act* protects _____ .
    a. current employees who become disabled
    b. former employees seeking to return to employment
    c. prospective employees with disabilities from job discrimination
    d. A and C

17. For an interview in a dental office, it is appropriate for a female interviewee to
    wear _____ .
    a. a business suit and low heels
    b. a dental assist uniform
    c. a fancy dress and jewelry
    d. informal clothing

18. Following the interview it is most appropriate to send _____ .
    a. a copy of your school or college transcript
    b. a follow-up thank-you letter
    c. flowers or other thank-you gift
    d. another copy of your résumé

19. A written document that clarifies the terms of employment is known as a/an _____ .
    a. contract
    b. employment agreement
    c. job description
    d. job offer

20. Stealing and the use of illicit drugs are examples of cause for _____ .
    a. probation
    b. salary reduction
    c. summary dismissal
    d. termination

21. A neat uniformed appearance includes _____ .
    a. a bow to keep hair tied back
    b. a wrist watch
    c. an association pin
    d. B and C

22. A chairside assistant should change into the uniform at _____ .
    a. home
    b. the office

23. An assistant employed by a dental school _____ .
    a. is considered to be part of the faculty
    b. is expected to conduct training seminars for the students
    c. works as a paid assistant to dental students
    d. A, B, and C

24. During the interview, it _____ appropriate for the applicant to ask questions about salary and benefits.
    a. is
    b. is not

25. Work experience is listed on the résumé with the _____ job first.
    a. best paying
    b. first
    c. most important
    d. most recent

Competency 36 - 1 *Being Interviewed for a Position as a Chairside Assistant*

Performance Objective: With the instructor or another student playing the role of the interviewer, the student will demonstrate interviewing for a position as a chairside assistant.

Important: Before the interview, the student will have prepared and submitted to the interviewer a letter of application and a résumé.

Note: The class discussion replaces the use of individual evaluators.

The applicant is Paula Graves:
Paula has recently graduated from a dental assisting program and is now a CDA. She is also a registered assistant in this state.

The interviewer is Mrs. Adams:
Mrs. Adams is the office manager and is in charge of hiring.
There is an opening in the practice for a chairside assistant.
Mrs. Adams really would prefer someone with more experience.

Check box if the step was performed correctly.

1. The applicant was dressed appropriately for an interview. As an alternative, she may describe appropriate dress. ❑

2. The applicant's letter of application was neat and contained the appropriate information. ❑

3. The applicant's résumé was well organized and professional in appearance. ❑

4. The applicant answered the interviewer's questions. ❑

5. The applicant asked appropriate questions. ❑

6. The applicant made a good, professional impression. ❑

7. At the end of the interview, the applicant thanked the interviewer. ❑

Notes:
Based on the information brought out during the interview, the class may wish to discuss whether or not this is a good job opportunity for Paula.
They might also want to discuss how they would feel about working with Mrs. Adams.

Dental Specialty Study Cards

(To use, remove the page from the workbook and separate the cards.)

Dental Public Health	**Endodontics**
Oral Pathology	**Oral and Maxillofacial Surgery**
Orthodontics	**Pediatric Dentistry**
Periodontics	**Prosthodontics**

Dental Specialty Study Cards

_____ is concerned with the etiology, diagnosis, prevention, and treatment of diseases and injuries of pulp and associated periradicular tissues.

_____ is concerned with preventing and controlling dental diseases and promoting dental health through organized community efforts.

_____ is concerned with the diagnosis and surgical and adjunctive treatment of diseases, injuries, and defects of the oral and maxillofacial region.

_____ is concerned with the nature of the diseases affecting the oral structures and adjacent regions.

_____ is primarily concerned with the preventive and therapeutic oral health care of children from birth through adolescence.

_____ is concerned with the supervision, guidance, and correction of all forms of malocclusion of the growing or mature dentofacial structures.

_____ is concerned with the maintenance of oral functions by the restoration of natural teeth and/or the replacement of missing teeth.

_____ is concerned with the diagnosis and treatment of disease of the supporting and surrounding tissues of the teeth.

Angle's Classification Study Cards

(To use, remove the page from the workbook and separate the cards.)

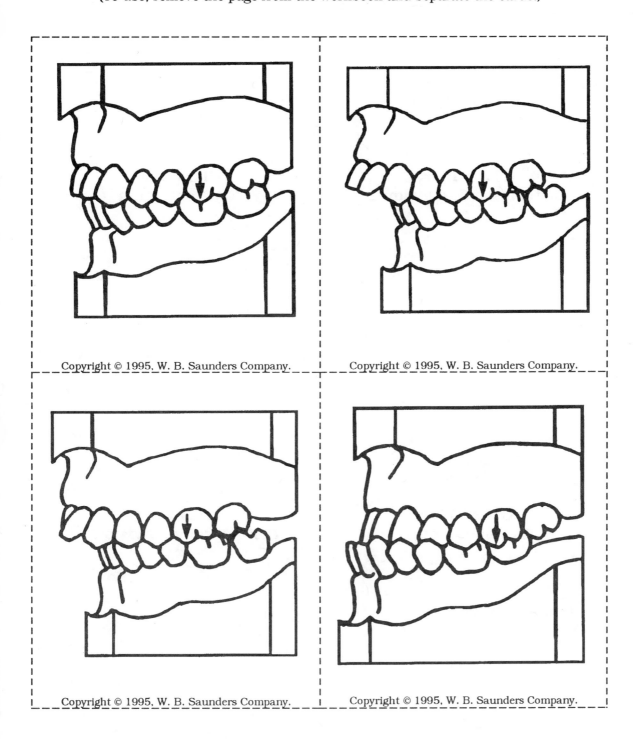

233

Class II, or
Distoclussion, division 1

Class I, or
Neutroclussion

Class III, or
Mesioclussion 1

Class II, or
Distoclussion, division 2

Dental Hand Instrument Study Cards (1)

(To use, remove the page from the workbook and separate the cards.)

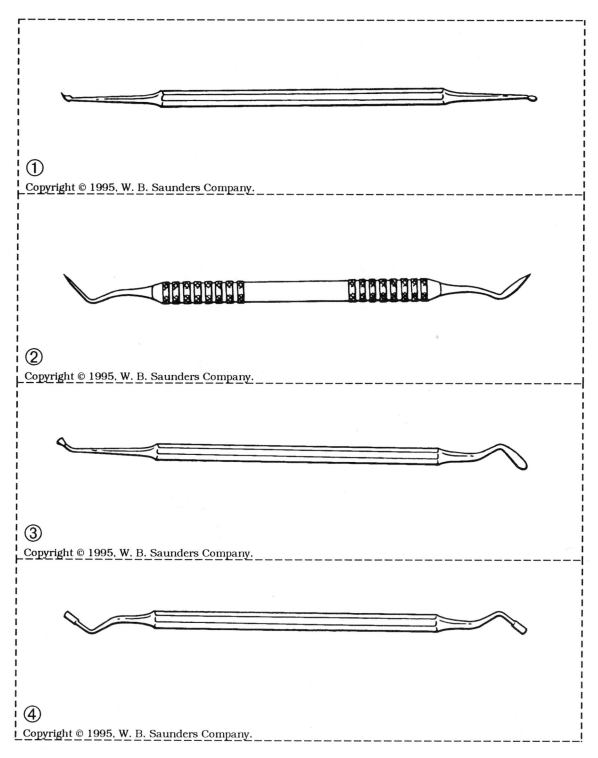

①

②

③

④

235

Discoid-cleoid carver

Hollenback carver

Woodson plastic filling instrument

Double-ended amalgam condenser

Dental Hand Instrument Study Cards (2)

(To use, remove the page from the workbook and separate the cards.)

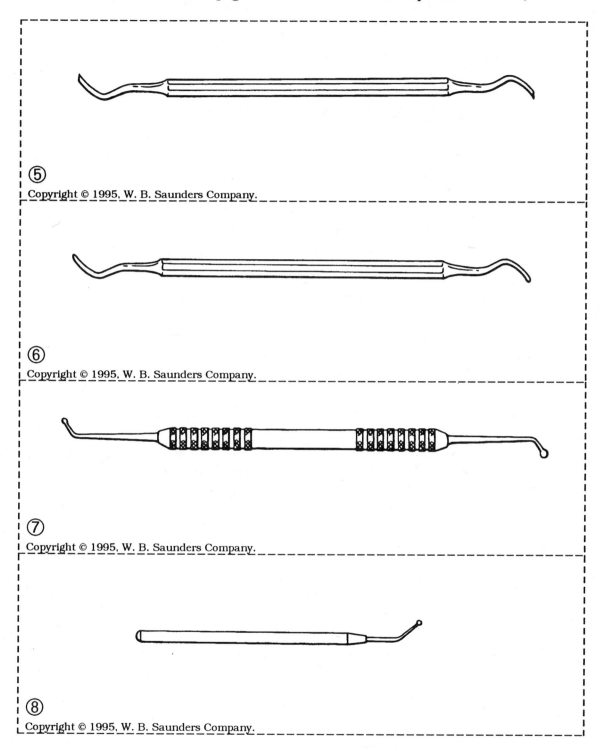

⑤

⑥

⑦

⑧

Gingival margin trimmer

Spoon excavator

Double-ended ball burnisher

Cavity liner applicator

Cavity Classification Study Cards

(To use, remove the pages from the workbook and separate the cards.)

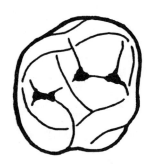

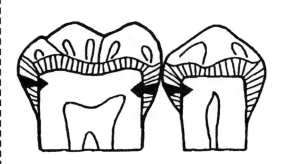

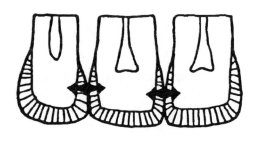

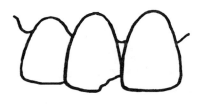

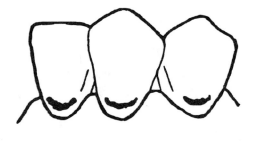

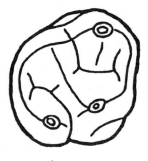

Class II
Posterior interproximal cavities

Class I
Pit and fissure cavities

Class IV
Anterior interproximal cavities
involving the incisal edge

Class III
Anterior interproximal cavities

Class VI
Worn or abraded incisal or
occlusal surfaces

Class V
Smooth surface or
cervical cavities